General Surgical Emergencies

An on-the-spot guide

James Hill

Published by the REMEDICA Group

REMEDICA Publishing Ltd, 32–38 Osnaburgh Street, London, NW1 3ND, UK
REMEDICA Inc, Tri-State International Center, Building 25, Suite 150, Lincolnshire, IL 60069, USA

E-mail: books@remedica.com
www.remedica.com

Publisher: Andrew Ward
In-house editors: Roisin O'Brien and Emma Hawkridge
Cover design: Tom Gordon

ISBN 1 901346 27 7
British Library Cataloguing-in Publication Data
A catalogue record for this book is available from the British Library

Printed and bound at Ajanta Offset & Packagings Ltd., India

General Surgical Emergencies

An on-the-spot guide

James Hill

Consultant General and Colorectal Surgeon
Department of Surgery
Manchester Royal Infirmary
Oxford Road
Manchester
M13 9WL
UK

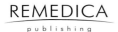

REMEDICA
publishing

LONDON • CHICAGO

Contributors

Mohammed Baguneid, MD, MRCS
Clinical Fellow in Vascular Surgery, Manchester Royal Infirmary

Richard Bowman, MD, BA, FRCA
Consultant Anesthetist, Manchester Royal Infirmary

James Hill, MD, ChM, FRCS
Consultant General and Colorectal Surgeon, Manchester Royal Infirmary

Ian MacLennan, MD, FRCS
Consultant General and Colorectal Surgeon, Manchester Royal Infirmary

Richard Napier-Hemy, MD, FRCS
Consultant Urological Surgeon, Manchester Royal Infirmary

Robert Pearson, MD, FRCS
Consultant General and Colorectal Surgeon, Manchester Royal Infirmary

Ajith Siriwardena, MD, FRCS
Consultant General and Hepatobiliary Surgeon, Manchester Royal Infirmary

Vince Smyth, MD, MChir, FRCS
Consultant Vascular Surgeon, Manchester Royal Infirmary

Foreword

This is a new presentation of basic surgical matters suitable for the novice surgeon. Such a book is needed because of the demise of the apprenticeship system of training which has pertained worldwide until recent changes in British surgery have substituted education for learning.

This book is essential reading for the new type of surgical trainee, for in addition to dealing with the many clinical situations the young surgeon may meet, it emphasizes the requirement for continuity of care and lays down rational rules as to how this may be achieved. It touches on guidelines, the responsibility of doctors and how to deal with interpersonal difficulties. The issues of delegation and consent are addressed.

The clinical section deals with the common emergency clinical presentations encountered in a busy general hospital and recognizes that this will include urology and vascular surgery as well as abdominal and colorectal problems. Such an approach is required as general surgery has become more subdivided into specialties; the patients, however, do not necessarily conform to those subdivisions.

The clinical section highlights the important elements of history, examination and investigation appropriate for the adequate assessment of the emergency patient. The pitfalls of management are illustrated by both examples of 'disaster scenarios' and by pointing out common errors. The book is both practical and detailed in the essentials of diagnosis and perioperative management. This leads to clear advice, much of which is admirable.

The last section of the book deals with the important topic of postoperative complications. This is a subject which the surgical trainee finds difficult and is a common source of delay and error. For this reason this is an especially valuable section.

Mr Hill is to be congratulated on this book which he has conceived and brought to fruition with his colleagues from Manchester Royal Infirmary. Study of this book will add valuable practical insight for any trainee, help to prevent errors and improve the standard of care given to patients.

Philip Schofield
Emeritus Professor of Surgery
Victoria University of Manchester

Contents

chapter 1

Organizational issues

James Hill

The role of the surgical resident is critically important in almost every general surgical emergency and many difficult situations that are faced can be made easier to deal with by good organization skills. These include establishing clear and regular communication with other members of the on-call team, namely the nursing staff, the theater staff, relatives and patients. All members of the on-call team should have a clear understanding of their responsibilities and they should make sure that they are working within the limits of their professional competence.

Communication

In most hospitals, the surgical resident is the first point of contact for the acute surgical patient. His or her duties include taking a history, examining the patient and deciding what the first-line investigations should be. The surgical resident will often be on duty with team members that he or she does not know, rather than those worked with on a regular basis. Adequate communication with the rest of the on-call team is therefore vital.

The surgical resident must know who is responsible for chasing up investigation results and making sure that these results are in the notes. Usually this is either the responsibility of the surgical resident or the house officer. It is also the responsibility of the surgical resident to ensure, when he or she goes off duty, that the person covering is provided with a written list of all admissions.

Senior staff should be contacted for:

- all patients who require surgery
- any patient requiring resuscitation or transfer to the high dependency unit (HDU) or the intensive care unit (ICU), together with patients transferred to the ICU from another hospital
- any patient with medico-legal implications, e.g. involvement with the police, aggrieved relatives or sudden deaths
- reasons of courtesy towards hospital staff
- patients with no clear diagnosis or progress

At the end of your period on call you must pass on details of patients that you have admitted to a member of the responsible consultant's team.

The following minimum information should be communicated:

- name, age and location of the patient
- primary diagnosis and general well-being of the patient
- actions you have taken or have planned
- results of initial investigations

It is much more reliable to write a list of these details as you go along rather than trying to remember them at 8 am the following morning.

Continuity of care

It is impossible for any one individual to carry the sole responsibility for continuity of care. The General Medical Council (GMC) advises doctors to, when off duty, ensure that arrangements are made for their patients' medical care, including effective hand-over procedures and clear communication between doctors. Continuity of care is an organizational matter for which the doctor has an ethical, but not a legal responsibility.

Delegation, accountability and independence

The surgical resident is responsible for all decisions and actions that he or she takes, along with any delegated to others. It is reasonable and sensible to delegate tasks to more junior staff, if they fall within their sphere of capability and if they have time to do them. Make sure that your instructions are clear. This makes life easier for you and the person performing the task.

For example "check Mr Smith's blood count" may be interpreted as:

- simply sending the blood sample off
- sending the blood sample off and knowing the result
- sending the blood sample off, knowing the result and writing the result in the notes
- sending the blood sample off, knowing the result, writing the result in the notes and telling you the result of the test
- all of the above and acting on the result

Being accountable means taking responsibility for tasks and decisions appropriate to your level of experience, keeping more senior members of the team informed about your activities and not performing tasks beyond your expertise and training.

When you carry out any duty, the GMC states you must "recognize and work within the limits of your professional competence". Similarly, when work is delegated, the individual delegating the work must "be sure that the person to whom you delegate the work is competent to carry out the procedure". The individual delegating the work remains responsible for the overall management of the patient.

An area of debate surrounds the definition of professional competence. To date no good definition exists, therefore, it is left to the judgment of the individual who is to perform the procedure and his or her supervising doctor. The onus is on the supervisor to ensure that the more junior doctor can perform the procedure safely. If the surgical resident has doubts about his or her own ability to perform a procedure, then there should be supervision.

For example, if you have performed sufficient appendectomies to carry out this procedure independently, and you have admitted a classic case of appendicitis, it is entirely reasonable to simply let a senior member of the team know the details of the case and when you plan to take the patient to theater. If the diagnosis is not clear or you are not confident to perform this procedure independently, you must let a senior team member know that you require his or her presence with you in theater at the start of the case.

Equally, if you have admitted a patient and you are unsure of the diagnosis and management, you need to discuss the case with a more senior member of the team.

Protocols and guidelines (how to react to them)

The consultant staff become extremely irritated when management guidelines that they have produced are ignored by junior staff. Find out what guidelines are available, obtain a copy, and if you feel your management would differ from that in the guidelines then discuss it with a more senior member of staff before enacting your management decision.

Locums

When working with a locum doctor you do not know, and who does not work regularly in the hospital, it is important to record carefully what has been communicated in the notes. If you are unhappy about what he or she is doing then discuss the case with the consultant. By the nature of the post, the locum may not know the hospital routines or procedures.

Difficult doctors

The GMC clearly states that the duties of a doctor must include "an adequate assessment of the patient's condition, based on the history and clinical signs, and if necessary an appropriate examination" and "referring the patient to another practitioner when indicated". If a patient is under the care of your team, there is no scope for debate about your responsibilities. If you ask another practitioner for an opinion, your view may differ from his or her view about the "when indicated" referred to in the guidelines, and about the necessity for the other practitioner seeing the patient and performing "an appropriate examination". What action can you take if the practitioner that you have asked to see "your" patient refuses to do so?

The following tactics are almost always rewarded:
- make it clear that you are requesting the other doctor to see your patient
- speak to a senior member of your team to ensure that they agree that the referral or request is appropriate and then speak to the unhelpful doctor again
- speak to a more senior member of the team to which the doctor you are seeking an opinion from belongs
- tell the unhelpful doctor that you are going to write in the notes that you have requested him or her for an opinion

Remember to try to resolve all disputes like this amicably. The doctor's mess is a happier place if this is achieved. The same strategies should be employed if you are trying to arrange blood tests or radiological investigations.

Consent

When obtaining consent, patients or relatives should be given a description of the natural history of the condition and the medical therapies that are available.

The nature of the procedure should be explained, when known preoperatively. In the emergency situation it is important to explain that the findings during operation and, therefore, the exact procedure undertaken, are not always predictable. Morbidity and mortality are higher than for equivalent elective procedures. This should be explained to patients and relatives (the latter particularly when the risks are high). In situations where formation of a stoma is possible, mention this specifically.

Special issues relating to consent are:

- patients under 16 years old cannot give written consent so a parent or legal guardian must sign the consent form
- unconscious patients cannot give consent and nor can anyone else give consent on their behalf. Speaking to the next of kin, explaining the consent issues to them and seeking their approval for the planned procedure are nevertheless a vital and necessary part of the patient's treatment. Prior discussion of these issues is important as this may be difficult if a life-threatening situation arises
- patients refusing consent are fortunately few and far between. If they are capable of reaching a sane and balanced judgment and you have been through the consent process you can do no more. If there are doubts about an individual's ability to make this decision, seek advice from the duty psychiatrists and where possible involve the patient's family. Always seek senior advice if this situation arises

Making a decision not to operate on a patient

The decision not to operate on a patient needs to be made at the consultant level, ideally by two consultants. There are a variety of scoring systems, such as the Acute Physiology And Chronic Health Evaluation (APACHE) II and the Physiological and Operative Severity Score for the enUmeration of Mortality and Morbidity (POSSUM), that predict postoperative morbidity and mortality. These symptoms were designed to allow retrospective analysis of relative outcomes and therefore should not be used to make decisions about the suitability of surgery for individual patients.

Even after extended periods of time in the ICU, there is a reasonable expectation of a return to the previous quality of life. This recovery can take weeks to months. The decision to operate is therefore based just as much on an assessment of the patient's existing quality of life and the natural history of the underlying disease process as it is on the predicted survival rate. The decision not to operate must involve the patient (if he or she is well enough) and the relatives.

Difficult patients

The patient who has suffered trauma, in association with intoxication, is a common clinical situation that the surgical resident must deal with.

Assessment of these patients is more difficult because:

- the patient is frequently uncooperative
- it is difficult to assess whether the examination findings are more related to the drug or drugs causing the intoxication or the injuries that have been sustained

Patients like this often engender feelings of irritation and anger, particularly if you are busy trying to accomplish many tasks. As the history may be incomplete and inaccurate, try to establish mechanisms of injury from accompanying persons, the police or paramedics. Basic information such as 'was the person unconscious at the scene?' or 'when did he or she regain consciousness?' will be useful. With trauma patients you should always try to predict the likelihood of significant injury. It is sensible to err on the side of overinvestigation, rather than to assume that the intoxication accounts for the clinical condition.

It is always important to remember that any patient who is seriously ill, especially when hypoxic, can be uncooperative. Satisfy yourself that the uncooperative patient is unwell by clinical examination and the appropriate physiological measurements, i.e. full blood count, urea and electrolytes, glucose, blood gases and electrocardiogram. Remember the risk of aspiration in any patient whose conscious level is reduced, whatever the reason may be. In these cases nurse in the lateral position.

Following these simple general rules avoids most of the management pitfalls that are otherwise regularly encountered. These apply to all the specific acute general surgical conditions described in the proceeding chapters.

chapter 2

Upper gastrointestinal emergencies

James Hill & Robert Pearson

Esophageal perforation

Spontaneous esophageal perforation and iatrogenic perforation of the esophagus are rare. The proposed mechanism of injury in spontaneous perforation is a sudden and large rise in esophageal pressure during vomiting that is sufficient to cause rupture. Unlike the rest of the gastrointestinal (GI) tract, the esophageal wall does not have a serosa, making it more vulnerable to this form of injury. The subsequent clinical course is determined by the size of the esophageal defect (the defect is a longitudinal tear). When there is a large tear in the esophageal wall, the mediastinum fills with gas and fluid from the stomach (see Figure 2.01). Over the next few hours, the mediastinal pleura ruptures and a left-sided pleural effusion and collection develops. The patient becomes rapidly septic (see Figure 2.02). If treated more than 24 hours after rupture, the degree of sepsis is such that morbidity and mortality increase significantly.

The defect in the esophagus is sometimes so small that only gas leaks into the mediastinum. Under these circumstances sepsis is much less likely to develop and presentation may be delayed for days or even weeks after the rupture.

Presentation

Spontaneous esophageal perforation classically presents with the acute onset of severe chest or upper abdominal pain after vomiting. The pain often radiates to the back and is so severe that a dissecting thoracic aneurysm is an important differential diagnosis. The pain is unremitting and is associated with pleuritic chest pain of increasing severity and shortness of breath. If the perforation is iatrogenic, the endoscopist or radiologist should recognize the injury when performing the procedure. If iatrogenic perforation is not recognized, the presentation varies from mild chest pain with surgical emphysema and a change in the voice due to free gas around the larynx (the patient sounds as if they are speaking having previously inhaled helium), to the rapidly progressive deterioration described above. Large amounts of free gas may be present because of air insufflation at the time of endoscopy. With iatrogenic perforations, the hole in the esophagus is usually at least the diameter of

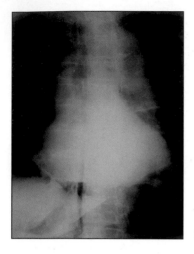

Figure 2.01 Esophageal rupture causing free gas within the mediastinum.

the instrument. On examination it is vital to feel for surgical emphysema in the tissues above the clavicle.

> **!** Crepitus is an early and reliable sign.

If crepitus is present assume that a perforation has occurred. The abdomen can be very tender and intraperitoneal perforation is often falsely suspected; a negative laparotomy has often been described. Look for systemic signs of sepsis and fluid at the left-lung base.

If you suspect esophageal rupture or perforation, arrange a plain chest x-ray (CXR) and a gastrografin swallow. Do not attempt to pass a nasogastric (NG) tube. Treatment with antibiotics should be initiated as soon as the diagnosis is suspected. Free gas in the mediastinum can be difficult to see, especially if you are not specifically looking for it (rather like the missing soft-tissue shadow on a CXR in a patient who has had a mastectomy). It is worth speaking to the radiologist prior to the test to inform him of your concerns regarding esophageal rupture. If there is no leak with gastrografin, repeating the test with barium is worthwhile as this is more sensitive for detecting small leaks.

Why is a contrast study necessary?

- to confirm the diagnosis – free mediastinal gas is not always a sign of esophageal rupture. It can occur after rupture of a lung bulla in which case a contrast study

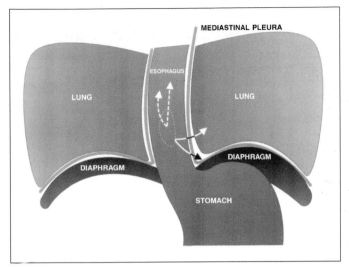

Figure 2.02 Line diagram showing the spread of sepsis (arrows) following esophageal rupture.

would be normal. In some cases, where a contrast study has not been done, surgical exploration has been performed unnecessarily

- to look at the anatomic site of leakage – the lower third on the left side is the most common site of leakage and spontaneous perforation (see Figure 2.03), but mid- and right-sided rupture have also been described. Iatrogenic perforations can occur at any site. It would be a disaster to perform a left thoracotomy if the leak is in the cervical esophagus

- to look at the size of the esophageal perforation – in a well patient, it may be safe to manage a small leak conservatively with broad-spectrum antibiotics and intravenous (IV) fluids, restricting oral fluids until the defect has closed. For larger perforations in patients with increasing sepsis, exposure of the affected esophagus and repair are required. Thoracotomy or exposure of the cervical esophagus is performed as appropriate. Iatrogenic perforations occurring during the management of esophageal carcinoma can be treated by insertion of a covered stent across the injury (see Figures 2.04)

Acute dysphagia

Total dysphagia is defined as the inability to swallow anything, including saliva. The acute management of this problem is straightforward. Admit the patient, rehydrate him or her and arrange a contrast study or upper GI endoscopy for the following day.

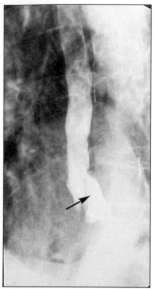
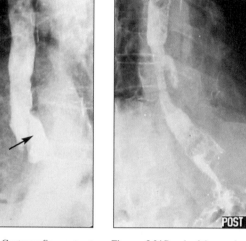
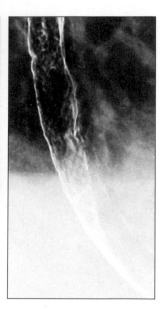

Figure 2.03 Gastrografin contrast study showing a leak from the lower third of the esophagus on the left side (the most common site of rupture).

Figures 2.04 Repair of the esophageal leak in Figure 2.03 treated with a covered esophageal stent: (a) the stent has not fully dilated and a small leak persists; (b) the stent has fully dilated and the leak has sealed.

Upper gastrointestinal hemorrhage

Blood loss from the upper GI tract occurs most commonly as a result of ulceration of the mucosa and erosion of the wall of blood vessels. Peptic ulcer disease is the cause of upper GI bleeding in 90% of cases, with 80% of these bleeds stopping spontaneously (see Figure 2.05). In general, the greater the depth of the ulcer, the greater the likelihood of erosion into a large vessel. The gastroduodenal artery running behind the duodenum, and the splenic artery behind the gastric antrum, are the most common large vessels involved.

Common patterns of bleeding

- ongoing bleeding with very low hemoglobin (Hb) levels and rapidly progressive shock, which is only partly responsive to resuscitation
- limited episodes of blood loss, temporary hypotension, moderate reduction in Hb levels with restoration of blood pressure (BP) after resuscitation
- single low volume bleed or 'coffee ground' vomitus with no hypotension and normal Hb levels

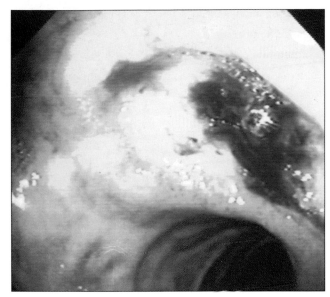

Figure 2.05 A bleeding duodenal ulcer.

Rapidly progressive shock is typically seen when there is erosion into a large vessel. Impressive volumes of blood can also be lost from large areas of superficial ulceration in the esophagus or in association with severe gastritis. The continued loss of 1 mL/minute will approximate to 1440 mL in 24 hours.

Bleeding in the absence of ulceration occurs with esophageal and gastric varices. Be aware of the existence of hemobilia (bleeding from the biliary tract). This is rare but should be suspected in a patient with upper GI bleeding showing a normal upper GI endoscopy.

Presenting features – questions to ask when a patient presents with upper GI bleeding

Q what is the estimated total volume of blood loss?

A ask patients, relatives or paramedics how much blood they saw

ask nursing staff to save any further hematemesis or melena for you to look at and to measure the blood loss and record it

Q has the patient had melena?

A the co-existence of hematemesis and melena usually indicates severe hemorrhage (a rough approximation is at least one-third of the circulating blood volume)

Q has the patient collapsed or lost consciousness as a result of the bleeding?

A this again indicates a more severe hemorrhage

Q are there typical symptoms of peptic ulcer disease?

A for example, epigastric pain, nausea, vomiting, sleep disturbance and periodicity

Q is there a previous history of peptic ulcers?

A this makes other causes of GI bleeding less likely

Q has the patient previously had definitive peptic ulcer surgery?

A there is a reduced risk of further life-threatening complications from peptic ulcer disease if the previous ulcer surgery included vagotomy or gastrectomy

Patient history (key questions)

Q is there a history of liver disease or excessive alcohol intake?

A think about varices, even though peptic ulcer disease is still more common in patients who are heavy alcohol consumers

Q is there a family history of peptic ulcer disease?

A this is surprisingly common

Q alcohol and smoking?

A smoking is probably of more importance in the development of peptic ulcers than heavy alcohol consumption

Q is the patient taking nonsteroidal anti-inflammatory agents or steroids?

A both increase the risk of developing a peptic ulcer

Q is the patient taking anticoagulants?

A clotting abnormalities may be the principal reason for the patient's bleeding

Q has the patient had aortic surgery?

A think about aortoenteric fistula

Q is there significant comorbidity?

A this is frequently present in elderly patients and important if surgery is being considered

Examination (key questions)

! The cause of GI bleeding in patients is often unresolved after examination.

Q are there any clues to the cause of the bleeding?

A look for signs of liver failure or abdominal scars

Q are there compensatory effects of bleeding on the cardiorespiratory system?

A look for pallor, sweating and/or cold clammy skin with peripheral vasoconstriction. A systolic BP of 120 mmHg may be significantly below the normal for an 85-year-old patient. Patients on β-blockers may not mount a tachycardic response to hypovolemia. Always count the respiratory rate. Hypovolemia increases the respiratory rate and respiratory effort thus increasing venous return to the heart.

Investigation (key questions)

Q what can we tell from the Hb level?

A firstly determine if the patient is anemic. Try to correlate the estimated total blood loss with the Hb level; this gives a better feel for how acute the bleeding has been. Some patients will present with a small bleed on top of chronic anemia. Remember that Hb is a measure of concentration (g/dL) so the severity of blood loss may not be fully reflected in the Hb level

Q is the urea level elevated?

A the urea level is elevated in upper GI bleeding because of the nitrogen load of digested blood. A urea/creatinine ratio greater than 100 is highly predictive of upper GI bleeding (urea and creatinine values in mmol/L)

Q is one venflon sufficient?

A usually yes, much more attention is given to patients having two venflons, than ensuring that patients are given sufficient fluid or blood. If there is evidence of severe bleeding insert two peripheral venflons; if there is ongoing hypotension a central line should be sited. (See Table 2.01.)

Q what should the initial infusate be?

A there has been a heated debate regarding crystalloid versus colloid as the initial infusate. If the BP is low it makes sense to give a plasma expander in the first instance. If this restores the blood pressure to normal it is perfectly acceptable to give crystalloid until blood is ready. Giving large volumes of colloid without blood can have a deleterious effect on clotting and should be avoided

Catheter	Volume (mL/minute)
Blue (22 Gauge)	31
Pink (20 Gauge)	55
Green (18 Gauge)	90
Gray (16 Gauge)	170
Brown/Orange (14 Gauge)	275

Table 2.01 Maximum volume of fluid that can be given via peripheral IV catheters.

Disaster scenario

An 85-year-old man is brought to the accident and emergency department.
Presenting complaint
- melena stools (x5/day)
- approximately 500–1000 mL in total

History of presenting complaint
- no previous ulcer

Previous history of illness
- ischemic heart disease

Examination
- pulse 86/minute, BP 120/80 mmHg, soft abdomen

Investigation
- Hb 8.9 g/dL, urea 11.5 mmol/L, creatinine 0.098 mmol/L
- clotting screen normal

Resuscitation
- single venflon (16 gauge-gray), with a 1 L crystalloid infusion over 8 hours

Further management
- nil by mouth with observation every 2 hours
- during first 24 hours after admission 2 units were transfused
- no further evidence of bleeding
- BP stable at 160/90 mmHg
- upper GI endoscopy arranged within 24 hours

Upper GI endoscopy
- lesser curve gastric ulcer with active bleeding and a suspicion of malignancy
- clot in the base of ulcer, not biopsied
- injected with 5 mL adrenaline solution (1/10,000), some oozing persists

Further developments
- the patient develops tachycardia and hypotension 24 hours later
- BP 90/70 mmHg associated with hematemesis (volume not ascertainable)
- Hb 8.5 g/dL
- after being reviewed by the surgical team an additional 2 units were transfused
- surgical team recommends further conservative therapy

Further developments
- a further episode of bleeding 72 hours after admission with hypotension developing

- Hb 8.5 g/dL, 4 units of blood given in total so far
- reviewed by the surgical team and in view of suspicion of malignancy no surgery was advised
- a further 2 units of blood were transfused

Final developments
- the patient has massive hematemesis and dies 96 hours after admission

Comment

At presentation, blood loss of this amount indicates a significant hemorrhage. At 85 years old with ischemic heart disease, a BP of 120/80 mmHg is likely to be abnormally low and this patient will tolerate hypotension poorly. The estimated blood loss and Hb level are in keeping with this patient having normal Hb prior to the bleed.

The urea/creatinine ratio is greater than 100 which indicates an upper GI hemorrhage.

Were the initial fluid replacements adequate? In this case almost certainly not. The patient has had an acute bleed and the fluid is being replaced at maintenance levels only. A unit of colloid over 1–2 hours would be very safe in this patient while waiting for blood results and cross-matching.

The initial 2 units of blood transfused was appropriate as there was no evidence of significant ongoing bleeding in the first 24 hours after admission. The transfusion should restore the Hb level to between 10–11 g/dL.

An endoscopy was arranged within an appropriate time as the patient was stable after admission. It is reasonable to defer biopsy in the presence of active bleeding. Any patient with a gastric ulcer should have a repeat gastroscopy with biopsy within a few weeks because of the risk of malignancy.

Is the residual oozing significant? Any residual bleeding is worrying and every effort should be made to bring it completely under control. If this is not successful the surgical team should be informed.

The tachycardia and hypotension, associated with hematemesis, 24 hours after admission was a clear indication of rebleeding. The only options at this stage are further therapeutic endoscopy, therapeutic angiography or laparotomy. The ulcer was clearly accessible for endoscopic treatment and therefore performing a repeat endoscopy was reasonable. If pursuing this approach, the endoscopy should be performed in the operating theater and should be followed by laparotomy unless the surgeon is confident that all bleeding has been controlled.

Surgery in this patient would carry a high risk, but in not operating the surgeon reviewing the case has erred on the side of hope above expectation. The patient only had a 2-unit transfusion but needed at least 2 further units of blood. The patient now met the criteria for surgical intervention.

The surgeon was fortunate and 72 hours after admission he was offered another chance to operate on the patient, who now had evidence of a second rebleed and required a 6-unit transfusion. The rebleeding is much more important than uncertainty about whether the lesion is malignant.

What was the risk associated with laparotomy? In elderly patients, urgent gastrectomy carries a mortality rate of up to 25%. The risk is less if no resection is performed and the bleeding vessel is simply under-run. It is vital to realize that the risk of doing nothing is much higher than the risk of a laparotomy. This is easily explained to the patient and relatives. In the presence of large volumes of GI blood loss the family are normally relieved that something is being done and will accept that major surgery in elderly patients is hazardous.

Q should the patient be transfused?

A in general aim for a Hb level between 10–11 g/dL and ensure that more blood is available in the event of further acute blood loss. A balance needs to be struck between the dangers of hypotension and the effects of transfusion. Hypotension may be particularly dangerous in elderly patients who may have underlying cardiovascular disease. Transfusion has an anticoagulant effect and raises the BP thus exacerbating the potential for further bleeding

Q is a NG tube necessary?

A surgeons tend to have strong views on this and they are equally likely to argue for and against a NG tube in patients with upper GI bleeding. Patients often tolerate the tube badly. Clotted blood cannot be aspirated and is often vomited around the tube. If the aspirate is clear it is unlikely that there is significant GI bleeding

> **!** All patients with upper GI bleeding require an upper
> GI endoscopy within 24 hours of admission.

Q when is endoscopy indicated out of hours?

A this is indicated if the patient remains hypotensive despite resuscitation or if the bleeding is persistent and of large volume. Whatever the organizational difficulties in arranging this, persistent hypotension (particularly in the elderly) and massive transfusion must be avoided

Q who should do the endoscopy?

A anyone who is competent in therapeutic endoscopy. Expert endoscopy improves the chances of nonoperative control of bleeding. Both the diagnosis and treatment are more difficult when there is blood in the stomach. Endoscopic indicators predictive of rebleeding are clots in the base of the ulcer, ooze or a visible or spurting vessel

Q what is the most effective treatment?

A when performed skillfully, injection sclerotherapy (with adrenaline or sclerosants) and heater probes; lasers and argon beam coagulators have similar success rates

Q should a gastric ulcer be biopsied?

A in the presence of bleeding it is reasonable to defer biopsy. Further endoscopy with biopsy should be performed when a patient has recovered from the acute episode

Perforated peptic ulcer

When an anterior gastric or anterior duodenal ulcer perforates (see Figure 2.06) through the full thickness of the bowel wall, enteric contents can pass into the peritoneal cavity. Over the first 6–8 hours the relatively sterile upper GI contents cause a chemical peritonitis. This then changes to a secondary bacterial infection leading to systemic sepsis. The suddenness of the perforation and the volume of escaping fluid mean that self-sealing of the perforation is not common. Posterior gastric perforation is rare and results in contamination of the lesser sac. If contained in the lesser sac an abscess forms. If there is leakage through the Foramen of Winslow, peritoneal irritation will result. Retroperitoneal duodenal perforation is a rare complication of endoscopic retrograde cholangiopancreatography; it usually resolves with conservative treatment.

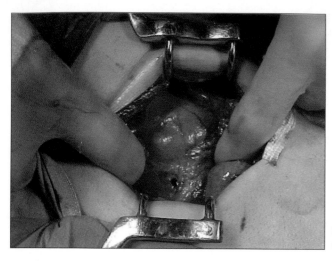

Figure 2.06 A typical perforated duodenal ulcer.

Presenting symptoms

When an anterior duodenal ulcer perforates, the onset of pain is typically sudden and starts in the epigastrium. The pain is severe and peritonitic in nature. As time passes (2–24 hours after perforation) the enteric contents produce a spreading peritonitis. The rate of spread depends on the size of the hole and the volume of enteric contents leaking into the peritoneal cavity. The initial spread of enteric contents may track down the right paracolic gutter with a similar extension of pain and tenderness. Vomiting is not prominent and shoulder tip pain is atypical in the early stages.

Around three-quarters of patients have had a previous history of suspected or proven peptic ulcer disease; therefore, obtaining this history is very important for the differential diagnosis. It is important to note that perforation is extremely rare in any patient on a therapeutic dose of proton-pump inhibitors. Acute complications of peptic ulcer disease can occur on maintenance doses of anti-ulcer drugs. A previous history of peptic ulcer disease is less common in elderly patients and those who perforate while taking nonsteroidal anti-inflammatory agents.

The findings on examination depend on the extent of spread of enteric contents and can therefore vary from localized epigastric peritonism to generalized peritonitis with a classical board-like rigidity. The extent of reduction in abdominal wall movement, bowel sounds and systemic signs also depends on the degree of peritoneal contamination. Diagnostic uncertainty decreases as time progresses. If there is a large

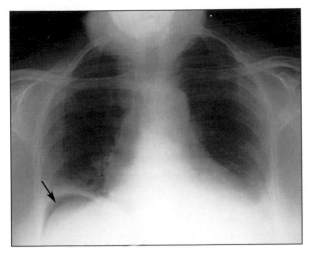

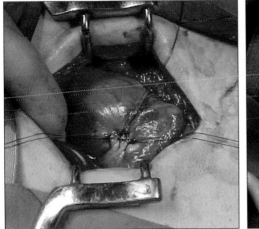

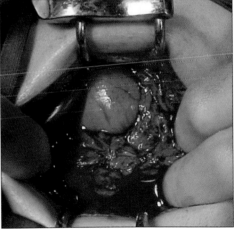

Figure 2.07 Free sub-diaphragmatic gas shown by x-ray. It is important to remember that one-third of patients display no free gas with a perforated peptic ulcer.

Figure 2.08 Repair of a perforated duodenal ulcer: (a) closure of the defect with interrupted absorbable sutures; (b) omental patch sutured over the repair.

amount of intraperitoneal free gas there may be loss of liver dullness on percussion, but this is an unreliable sign.

Although the morbidity and mortality will in general increase with the length of the period of peritoneal contamination, if you see a patient in the early stages after a perforation without free intraperitoneal gas on the erect CXR, then you (or indeed the higher surgical trainee or consultant) may well be unable to make the diagnosis with sufficient confidence to recommend laparotomy. This is not a problem as long as you make sure that the patient is reviewed, by yourself, in the next 2–3 hours. If the patient has a free perforation, the symptoms and signs will have increased and diagnostic uncertainty decreases.

Investigation

! An erect CXR will show no evidence of free gas in one-third to a half of cases.

If free gas is present, then an intra-abdominal viscus must have perforated. If fit enough, the patient should be resuscitated and prepared for laparotomy (see Figure 2.07).

Management

- oxygen 10 L/minute (unless the patient has chronic obstructive airways disease)
- resuscitation with IV fluid to achieve a urine output of 50 mL/hour or greater
- NG tube to minimize further peritoneal contamination
- broad-spectrum IV antibiotics to guard against enteric organism invasion
- opiate analgesia and anti-emetics
- consent – since the introduction of proton-pump inhibitors, vagotomy is virtually never performed. The patient can be told that the operation usually involves simply closing the hole (see Figure 2.08). If the defect is in the stomach then partial gastrectomy may be necessary. Remember to point out the uncertainty principle. You can never entirely remove the possibility that you will perform a negative laparotomy

chapter 3

Pancreatico–biliary problems

James Hill & Ajith Siriwardena

Acute cholecystitis

Acute cholecystitis is defined as an acute inflammation of the gallbladder, and is one of the most frequently encountered acute surgical conditions. In a survey of 10,682 patients with acute abdominal pain, 1005 (9.7%) were shown to have acute cholecystitis*. Gallstones are the principal cause of the condition. When a stone impacts in Hartmann's pouch or the cystic duct, the obstructed gallbladder distends and becomes tense. Normal emptying of the gallbladder is prevented and biliary stasis within this organ produces an environment that encourages bacterial growth. Traditionally it has been taught that the episode is resolved when the stone in Hartmann's pouch becomes disimpacted and the gallbladder is decompressed.

The life-threatening complications associated with acute cholecystitis are a result of bacterial proliferation; such complications are empyema, gallbladder perforation and necrotizing cholecystitis. The latter two conditions are uncommon because the gallbladder (unlike the appendix) has a good blood supply and is usually thick-walled from a previous chronic inflammation. The organisms most frequently associated are *Escherichia coli*, klebsiella and enterococci.

Presentation
The typical presentation is a history of right upper quadrant abdominal pain. There may have been a background of similar episodes triggered by the ingestion of fatty food. The pain may radiate around to the back and also be felt in the shoulder tip (the diaphragm is innervated by C3, C4 and C5, which are represented cutaneously over the shoulder). Typically, the pain is exacerbated by movement or coughing. Nausea and vomiting are usual and the patient may have noticed the presence of jaundice.

On examination, it is important to exclude septic shock or jaundice. The patient is likely to have a fever. Careful inspection is required to exclude scars of previous

---

* de Dombal FT. Diagnosis of acute abdominal pain. Second edition. Edinburgh: Churchill Livingstone, 1991.

surgery (in particular those of previous laparoscopic cholecystectomy). On palpation there should be evidence of localized guarding and peritoneal irritation in the right upper quadrant. The patient may elicit Murphy's sign. This is displayed as tenderness in the right upper quadrant during palpation that is made worse by the patient breathing in. This pain is thought to be due to the inflamed gallbladder moving down onto the examining hand. An acutely obstructed and distended gallbladder with adherent omentum can sometimes be palpated.

Investigation

The diagnosis of acute cholecystitis is suggested by the co-existence of right upper quadrant pain, peritoneal signs in this region, a raised temperature, and an elevated white blood cell (WBC) count. A differential diagnosis of acute peptic ulcer disease and acute pancreatitis must be taken into consideration. Baseline tests must, therefore, include an erect chest x-ray (CXR), as well as a plain abdominal film and a measurement of serum amylase.

An abdominal ultrasound scan is the investigation of choice. In practice, it is advisable to ensure that all the baseline tests have been performed (and the results known!) before proceeding with the scan. Initial efforts should be directed at making the diagnosis with reasonable certainty and ruling out other acute pathologies. Once this has been done, a decision needs to be taken regarding when the scan will be performed. In a stable patient with localized signs, the diagnosis on clinical grounds can be made with a reasonable degree of confidence and the ultrasound can be requested as an addition to the following day's list of scans in the radiology department. In situations where the patient is acutely ill with signs of both localized peritonitis and systemic 'toxicity', it is wise to consider an urgent ultrasound scan. This may require discussion between a more senior surgeon and radiologist.

An abdominal ultrasound scan will confirm the diagnosis of acute cholecystitis by demonstrating gallstones in a thick-walled gallbladder. The scan may also show pericholecystic fluid. The ultrasonographer should also comment on the diameter of the common bile duct (normally under 1 cm) and on the presence or absence of intrahepatic duct dilatation.

Biochemical liver function tests (LFTs) and a clotting screen complete the routine investigations in a patient with this condition. Blood cultures are worthwhile if the temperature rises above 38°C.

Management

> - intravenous (IV) crystalloid to replace fluid loss by vomiting and loss of normal intake
> - IV antibiotics to cover Gram-negative organisms
> - analgesia and anti-emetics; pethidine is recommended as it causes less spasm of the sphincter of Oddi than other opiates

The treatment of acute cholecystitis has evolved considerably in recent years. Two randomized trials of early versus late laparoscopic cholecystectomy have established that the acutely inflamed gallbladder can be safely removed laparoscopically. The practicalities of carrying out cholecystectomy in an emergency operating theater mean that the delayed surgery option is often selected.

If the clinician elects for delayed surgery then the patient has to be monitored with the expectation that there will be clinical improvement in response to treatment.

In situations where the focal signs persist, the patient may have an empyema (pus within the gallbladder) (see Figure 3.01), or more seriously, an infarcted necrotic gallbladder (see Figure 3.02). The typical picture of empyema of the gallbladder is a swinging pyrexia, tachycardia, static or worsening abdominal pain, and static or increasing abdominal tenderness.

Unresolving acute cholecystitis is frequently encountered. There are two main treatment options. Firstly, ultrasound-guided percutaneous cholecystostomy (insertion of a drain into the gallbladder) can be carried out. This is a relatively simple procedure and often gains valuable time in a patient who is seriously ill. It is important to remember that if the gallbladder is necrotic, it can still perforate despite the cholecystostomy tube, so the patient needs regular assessment until the acute sepsis has settled. The cholecystostomy tube is usually left *in situ* once it has been inserted as removal leaves the patient exposed to the risk of biliary peritonitis. A cholecystogram can be carried out through the cholecystostomy tube to confirm that there is free passage of contrast through the cystic duct into the common bile duct. The surgeon can then proceed with interval laparoscopic cholecystectomy as planned.

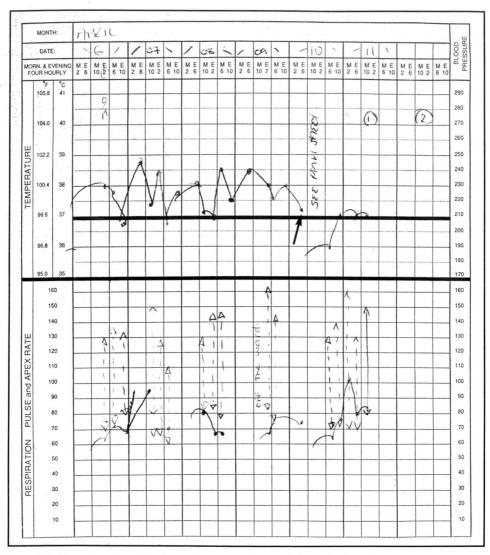

Figure 3.01 Temperature chart of a patient with empyema. The arrow indicates the time of surgery.

The alternative treatment for unresolving cholecystitis is to proceed to surgery. This is selected in younger patients without comorbidity. Although some surgeons would opt for an 'open' cholecystectomy in this situation, there is little to be lost by having a trial laparoscopic cholecystectomy, provided that the patient is aware that there is an increased chance of conversion to open-operation.

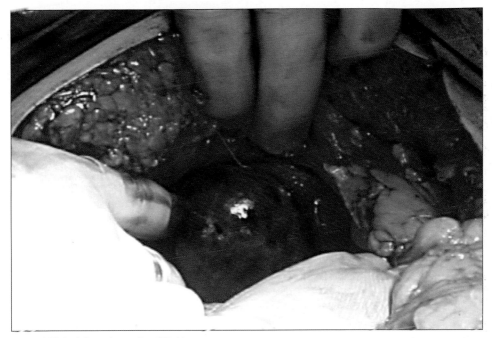

Figure 3.02 An infarcted necrotic gallbladder.

Biliary colic

Biliary colic is caused by a stone obstructing the neck of the gallbladder. The pathogenesis of biliary colic is identical to that of acute cholecystitis, with the only difference in clinical terms being less evidence of inflammation. To make a diagnosis of biliary colic, there should be a typical history of right upper quadrant pain, no signs of peritonitis, and the patient should be afebrile with a normal WBC count. The presence of abdominal signs, fever or elevated WBC levels all point towards acute cholecystitis.

In terms of practical management there is probably little to be gained by spending a great deal of effort distinguishing between the two conditions. With both, the gallbladder is obstructed with stones causing inflammation. In current practice, it seems sensible to establish the diagnosis by an ultrasound scan and then plan a definitive treatment strategy.

An important practical point is that the surgical resident will not usually have the benefit of access to ultrasound scanning while the patient is in casualty. Although it is tempting to discharge a patient with biliary colic, it is important to bear in mind that no diagnosis has been established. Therefore, in practice, admission to hospital followed by an in-patient ultrasound scan will help to confirm the condition and allow the development of a rational treatment plan.

Acute acalculous cholecystitis

In acalculous cholecystitis there is inflammation of the gallbladder in the absence of an obstructing stone. Increasingly, this is recognized as a manifestation of an ischemic process. The condition is principally seen in the intensive care unit (ICU) in patients with multiple system illness. From the point of view of the surgical resident, it is not uncommon to be called to an intensive therapy unit to give an opinion on a patient with fever and evidence of sepsis, where the common extra-abdominal causes (chest infection, urinary infection and line sepsis) have been ruled out. These patients will often be ventilated and thus unable to complain of abdominal pain but there may be signs of abdominal tenderness and unexplained deterioration in LFTs (be aware that both parenteral nutrition and antifungal therapy will interfere with LFTs). The diagnosis can be confirmed by an ultrasound scan and the condition can be treated by percutaneous cholecystostomy. Occasionally, cholecystectomy is required if the signs fail to resolve.

Cholangitis

Cholangitis is the clinical syndrome resulting from infection in an obstructed biliary tree. Classically, patients with cholangitis present with a high temperature, rigors (uncontrollable shaking) and jaundice (Charcot's triad). The two most common causes are obstruction of the distal common bile duct by a stone or a blocked endobiliary stent. Cholangitis frequently leads to bacteremia and septicemia.

The role of the surgical resident is to make the initial diagnosis, carry out basic tests and resuscitative maneuvers, and to inform senior colleagues of the situation.

Investigation
Following ultrasound scanning, the principal investigation is endoscopic retrograde cholangiography or ERC (usually referred to as endoscopic retrograde cholangiopancreatography [ERCP] because of the addition of a pancreatogram, which is not necessary in patients with cholangitis). ERC is carried out using a side-viewing fiberoptic endoscope. A clotting screen must be checked prior to ERC

and prophylactic antibiotics should be prescribed in the presence of an obstructed biliary tree. The doctor obtaining consent for ERC must inform the patient of the small risk of post-ERCP acute pancreatitis.

In addition to confirming the cause of cholangitis, ERC is the method of choice for removing the obstructing stone or blocked stent. If endoscopic access fails, the obstructed biliary tree can be decompressed by percutaneous insertion of an external biliary drain under ultrasound guidance.

A practical problem, which is often encountered, is the management of the patient who presents with cholangitis at weekends or in the absence of an endoscopist skilled in ERCP. In these situations, the initial resuscitation and diagnosis should proceed as outlined above. If the patient has presented at a weekend a combination of IV fluids and IV antibiotics will usually improve the situation until an endoscopist is available. If the problem is that the endoscopist is away, the patient should be stabilized and then transferred to another hospital for ERCP. The absence of an endoscopist on site is not an indication for surgical intervention.

Management

> - IV crystalloid to replace fluid loss by vomiting and loss of normal intake
> - IV antibiotics to cover Gram-negative organisms
> - analgesia and anti-emetics
> - baseline investigations include a full blood count (FBC), urea and electrolytes (U&E), LFTs, a clotting screen and blood cultures. A plain abdominal x-ray may confirm the presence of an endobiliary stent and an ultrasound scan may confirm dilatation of the common bile duct

It should be noted that cholangitis is principally a clinical diagnosis. Ultrasound may be insufficiently accurate to demonstrate extrahepatic duct obstruction caused by a gallstone impacted at the distal end of the common bile duct.

Acute pancreatitis

Acute pancreatitis is defined as an acute inflammation of the pancreas with variable involvement of remote organ systems. The current classification of acute pancreatitis was standardized at the Atlanta consensus conference in 1992. As a result, the nomenclature for describing acute pancreatitis is now simplified and relates to practical definitions of the disease.

> ❗ Acute pancreatitis is defined as either mild or severe.

Mild acute pancreatitis is a self-limiting illness characterized by the absence of organ dysfunction. In contrast, severe acute pancreatitis is characterized by the development of multiple organ dysfunction. There is a greater likelihood of severe pancreatitis if there is death of pancreatic tissue (pancreatic necrosis).

The role of the surgical resident in acute pancreatitis is:
- to make the diagnosis
- to exclude common differential diagnoses, in particular acute intestinal ischemia
- to stratify disease severity
- to ensure adequate fluid resuscitation
- to ensure adequate oxygenation
- to ensure adequate monitoring
- to inform senior colleagues of the case

Unit protocols may exist which must be followed regarding the use of prophylactic antibiotics, prophylactic anti-acid secretary medication, and low-dose heparin to prevent thromboembolic complications. Patients admitted to the high dependency unit (HDU) will normally have a central venous line inserted to monitor the central venous pressure. Although there is no evidence to disagree with this practice, there is a suggestion that line sepsis, resulting from this early central line, is a common cause of infection and pancreatic necrosis.

Diagnosis
Typically the patient presents with a history of rapid onset, severe epigastric pain. The pain usually radiates to the back and may be relieved by sitting up. Early and severe vomiting should always alert you to a possible diagnosis of pancreatitis.

On examination, the patient may be shocked. There may be a tinge of scleral jaundice. On abdominal inspection, there may be flank bruising resulting from the release of proteolytic enzymes into the retroperitoneum around the flanks (Grey Turner's sign). An important note of caution is that Grey Turner's sign can be closely mimicked by patients with flank bruising as a result of over-warfarinization. These patients may also have a raised serum amylase level. This diagnosis may be distinguished from that of acute pancreatitis when a normal pancreas is revealed by computed tomograph (CT) scan and a grossly prolonged prothrombin time is observed. Also, be aware of flank bruising that results from retroperitoneal rupture of an abdominal aortic aneurysm.

> ! Where there is diagnostic difficulty, contrast CT scanning is the single most useful test to establish the correct diagnosis.

Baseline tests for the diagnosis of acute pancreatitis must include the following:
- FBC
- serum U&E
- blood glucose
- serum amylase
- erect CXR
- plain abdominal x-ray
- electrocardiogram

Differential diagnosis
- acute peptic ulcer or perforated peptic ulcer
- acute cholecystitis
- acute myocardial infarcation
- acute intestinal ischemia

Stratifying disease severity
Once the diagnosis has been made, it is worthwhile carrying out severity stratification using either the Imrie (Glasgow) criteria or the Acute Physiology And Chronic Health Evaluation (APACHE) II score. The Ransom score is not frequently used as it refers to a North American population with alcohol as the dominant etiology. It is also difficult to estimate some parameters that are required for the calculation of Ransom, e.g. fluid sequestration.

A severe attack, using the modified Glasgow criteria for severity prediction in acute pancreatitis, is predicted by the presence of three or more positive criteria:
- arterial oxygen tension (pO_2) less than 8.0 kPa
- albumin less than 32 g/L
- serum calcium less than 2.0 mmol/L
- WBC count greater than 15×10^9/L
- aspartate aminotransferase greater than 200 U/L
- lactate dehydrogenase greater than 600 U/L
- blood glucose greater than 10 mmol/L (in the absence of diabetes)
- blood urea greater than 16 mmol/L

Fluid resuscitation, oxygenation and monitoring

Mild pancreatitis

If mild pancreatitis (less than three positive criteria) is predicted the following action should be taken:

- admit to the main ward
- IV crystalloid to maintain a urine output of 50–100 mL/hour
- maintain sodium (Na+) and potassium (K+) values in the normal range
- ensure that an accurate fluid balance chart is recorded
- maintain a pO_2 greater than 80 mmHg with oxygen supplementation
- insert a nasogastric (NG) tube if there is vomiting, nil by mouth
- control pain with pethidine (avoid morphine as it contracts the sphincter of Oddi)

Monitor

At the very least, make sure that the heart rate, blood pressure (BP), urine output and oxygen saturation levels are monitored. Check FBC, U&E, LFTs, and calcium, magnesium, glucose and amylase levels daily until the patient is stable. An ultrasound scan helps to confirm the diagnosis but be aware that abdominal distension with gas will affect the quality of the examination.

Severe pancreatitis

If severe pancreatitis is predicted (three or more criteria) the following action should be taken:

- admit to HDU or ICU
- insert a urinary catheter
- insert a central venous pressure line
- insert an arterial line

Monitor

The aims of treatment are the same as those for the ward care patient but the measures taken to achieve this may be more involved. For example, to maintain pO_2 levels, high-flow oxygen and continuous positive airway pressure (CPAP) may be required. An adult with acute severe pancreatitis will often require up to 5 L of fluid in 24 hours. Blood tests should also be carried out as with mild pancreatitis.

> **!** All patients with severe pancreatitis require an urgent CT scan with IV contrast to look for areas of non-enhancement in the pancreas.

Maintain a urine output of approximately 50 mL/hour. Most patients with acute pancreatitis do not require a NG tube in the early stages of the illness, but NG aspiration will help if persistent vomiting is a problem. Make sure that blood gases are checked and that the patient receives supplemental oxygen.

> ! There is always the risk that mild pancreatitis will develop into severe pancreatitis.

Danger Signs
- increasing abdominal pain and distension
- increasing respiratory rate
- persistent pyrexia and tachycardia
- hemoglobin (Hb) less than 10 g/dL
- platelets less than 50/mm^3
- WBC less than 3×10^9/L or persistently above the normal range
- abnormal clotting
- amylase not falling by day 3 to 50–70% baseline
- jaundice (consider endoscopic sphincterotomy)

What to do if danger signs are present:
- transfer to HDU or ICU
- urgent CT scan with IV contrast

Patients with acute severe pancreatitis due to gallstones may benefit from early ERC. At present, there appears to be some confusion about whether this should be performed. This decision is probably one for the senior team clinician to make. However, it is the responsibility of the surgical resident to make sure that LFTs are done and that an ultrasound scan is booked. If an ERC is planned, the surgical resident must also ensure that a clotting screen has been performed.

The ongoing management of severe acute pancreatitis, including the detection and management of local and regional pancreatic complications, is beyond the scope of this book.

chapter 4

Small bowel problems
Robert Pearson & James Hill

Small bowel obstruction

The cardinal features of intestinal obstruction are:

- colicky abdominal pain
- vomiting
- abdominal distension
- absolute constipation (no flatus or stool)

Presenting symptoms

The most common causes of small bowel obstruction are adhesions, hernias and malignancy. Presenting features depend on the location of the obstruction. The lower the obstruction the greater the distension will be. The higher the obstruction the greater the vomiting will be.

As soon as there is an obstruction, the patient experiences colicky abdominal pain which lasts for 1–2 minutes; this returns after an interval of several minutes. It is maximal around the umbilicus but is experienced throughout the abdomen. The peristalsis persists for 48 hours to several days. After this time, left untreated, peristalsis decreases until the bowel becomes flaccid and paralyzed. At this point, even when obstruction persists, pain improves or disappears; this is true unless there is strangulation. The vomitus consists of partly digested food and bile. With increasing stasis and bacterial overgrowth, brown offensive feculent (not fecal) fluid is seen (see Figure 4.01). The bowel below the obstruction functions normally and intestinal contents below the obstruction will be evacuated. Giving an enema can therefore be misleading.

Key questions that the surgical resident should bear in mind

Does the patient have a small bowel obstruction?
If the cardinal features described above are present then there is little doubt about the diagnosis of intestinal obstruction. On examination look for potential causes of the obstruction. Carefully feel hernial orifices. Remember that a Richter's type femoral

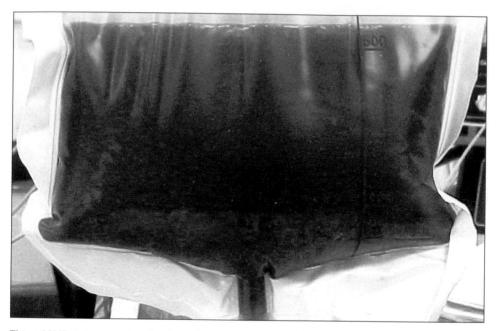

Figure 4.01 Typical nasogastric aspirate in a patient with small bowel obstruction; note the debris in the lower part of the drainage bag.

hernia may be small and difficult to palpate and that elderly patients are frequently not aware that there is a lump in their groin (see Figure 4.02). All patients who have had a laparotomy are at risk of adhesional obstruction. Confirm that the abdomen is distended, look for visible peristalsis (this can sometimes be stimulated by 'flicking' the abdominal wall) and listen for obstructed bowel sounds.

> **!**   Much can be determined from a plain abdominal x-ray.

Is the small bowel dilated?
Use the rule of thumb, i.e. if the small bowel diameter is greater than the distal phalanx of your thumb then the small bowel is dilated (see Figure 4.03).

Is there any large bowel gas or distension?
Look for the haustral markings of the colon. Colonic gas is only present in early or partial small bowel obstruction. The presence of small bowel and colonic distension indicates that the patient has either pseudo-obstruction or mechanical colonic obstruction with an incompetent ileo-cecal valve.

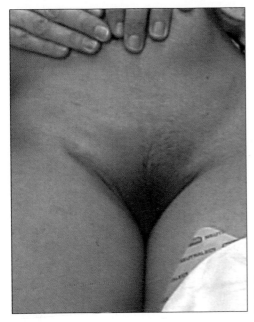

Figure 4.02 A patient with small bowel obstruction caused by an asymptomatic femoral hernia. Always examine the groin of a patient with a small bowel obstruction.

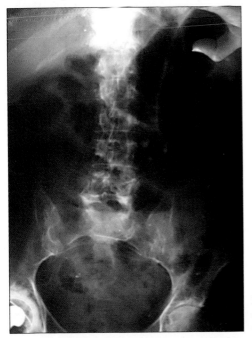

Figure 4.03 Typical x-ray of a patient with a small bowel obstruction. The rule of thumb indicates a distended small bowel.

Is an erect abdominal x-ray required?
This has now gone out of vogue. If there is clear evidence of small bowel obstruction on the supine view the erect x-ray adds little. If you are unsure about the supine view obtain an erect x-ray to look for fluid levels.

Is there gas in the biliary tree?
Remember to look specifically for gas in the biliary tree. This is seen in gallstone ileus, after endoscopic retrograde cholangiopancreatography with sphincterotomy and after anastomosis between the bile duct and duodenum (see Figure 4.04). The small bowel obstruction observed with gallstone ileus typically relents then exacerbates.

What is the extent of dehydration?
Dehydration results from a combination of loss of normal oral intake, fluid losses in the vomitus and fluid sequestered in the distended intestine. Examination findings of loss of skin turgor and sunken eyes give an impression of the severity of dehydration; however, these are imprecise. Better estimates are obtained by measuring urea and electrolytes (U&E) and the hematocrit but even the results of these tests do not tell how much fluid to administer. The extent of dehydration can only accurately be determined by measuring the central venous pressure (CVP) or the left atrial pressure. The simplest method is to measure hourly urine output and give sufficient fluid to maintain an output of 50 mL/hour or greater. The infused fluid should be normal saline or physiological Ringer's lactate. If the potassium level is low, potassium must be added to the infusion fluid. Even if potassium is normal it should be checked after a few hours as potassium levels will fall during resuscitation.

> **!** All patients with intestinal obstruction require a nasogastric (NG) tube. This reduces abdominal distension and the risk of aspiration.

Are there any clinical features to suggest actual or impending intestinal ischemia?
Features of strangulation are continuous unremitting pain and severe pain only partially relieved or unrelieved by opiate analgesics. On examination, the degree of tachycardia, tenderness, localized tenderness and peritonism are the most important signs to look for. Determine whether dilated bowel loops seen on x-ray correspond to the area of maximal tenderness (see Figure 4.05). It is usually a combination of these features rather than a single finding that suggests ischemia. If the small bowel is grossly dilated the risk of perforation and ischemia are high. If there is evidence of

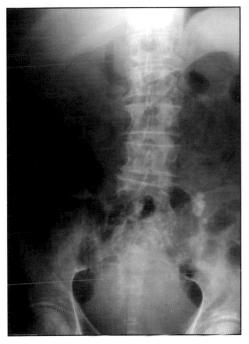

Figure 4.04 Gas in the biliary tree is rare and not seen unless specifically looked for.

closed loop obstruction, an urgent laparotomy is required as the risk of strangulation and perforation is greater. A substantially elevated white blood cell (WBC) count (greater than 20×10^9/L) indicates that ischemia is more likely, but note that a normal WBC count does not exclude the disease.

If there is a possibility that ischemia is present, an urgent laparotomy is required. In this case, resuscitation will need to be more rapid and should therefore be guided by central monitoring. This is best carried out in the high dependency unit (HDU), the intensive care unit or the anesthetic room. In the absence of any clinical suspicion of ischemia, it is appropriate to manage the patient with NG aspiration and intravenous (IV) rehydration. Should features of ischemia develop, an urgent laparotomy is required. Otherwise, the length of time it is reasonable to treat the patient conservatively is judged on the length of the preceding history and the completeness of the obstruction. If the patient is admitted with a 5-day history of obstruction, the test of conservative treatment has been done at home and resolution without surgery is highly unlikely. As a generalization, in complete obstruction, if there is no sign of improvement after 24 hours of conservative therapy then laparotomy should

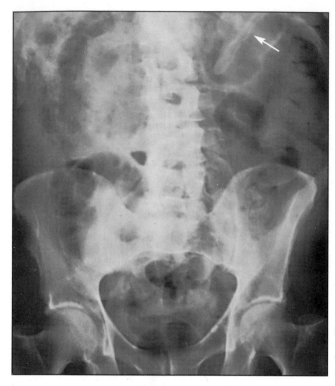

Figure 4.05 Small bowel ischemia is difficult to diagnose. It is suspected when edematous small bowel loops are seen (arrow).

be performed. If the patient has not had previous intra-abdominal surgery (and therefore has no surgery-induced adhesions) there is less likelihood of the obstruction settling. Clearly, if a cause for the obstruction is identified, such as a hernia, surgery is necessary.

Partial or subacute small bowel obstruction

The typical presentation is colicky abdominal pain with vomiting and distension but without absolute constipation. Examination findings are often non-specific and plain x-rays typically show a few dilated small bowel loops; there is no urgent need for laparotomy. Under these circumstances, a computed tomograph (CT) scan with oral contrast or a small bowel enema are the best lines of investigation. Should one be equivocal, then the other investigation is worthwhile.

Disaster scenario

A 28-year-old man is admitted at 9 pm with a 24-hour history of colicky abdominal pain, vomiting, distension and absolute constipation. Previously, a subtotal colectomy had been performed. On admission he has severe continuous abdominal pain, not adequately controlled with intramuscular morphine.

Examination
- pulse 110/minute
- blood pressure (BP) 120/80 mmHg
- generally tender abdomen with rebound tenderness around the umbilicus
- moderate distension
- obstructed bowel sounds

Investigation
- distal small bowel obstruction confirmed by x-ray
- hemoglobin 14.6 g/dL
- WBC 21x10^9/L

The surgical resident diagnoses small bowel intestinal obstruction and initiates conservative management with IV fluid and a NG tube overnight. The same surgical resident reviews him 2 hours later and administers IV morphine because the pain is uncontrolled. He is next reviewed at 9 am when he is in severe pain, with a BP of 100/60 mmHg, a pulse of 130/minute and a rigid abdomen.

Laparotomy reveals adhesional obstruction of the small bowel with infarction from the ileostomy to proximal jejunum. The infarcted intestine was excised and the patient survived but required lifetime parenteral nutrition.

Comment

Classical symptoms, such as the continuous and severe nature of the pain (not even controlled by IV opiates), associated tenderness, peritonism and a raised WBC level, all make ischemia extremely likely. A decision to perform laparotomy should have been made at the initial assessment and the need for laparotomy was even more certain when IV opiate could not control the pain. The patient needed a laparotomy as soon as he could be made fit for a general anesthetic.

Hernias

When intestine becomes trapped acutely within a hernia sac it may:

- reduce spontaneously
- remain incarcerated and viable
- become obstructed and remain viable
- become strangulated

The narrowing, edema and angulation caused when the intestine is trapped are often sufficient to obstruct the lumen and a sequelae of intestinal obstruction follows. If the pressure in the intestinal wall becomes higher than the venous pressure, venous return is impaired increasing the pressure in the intestinal wall further. The increased pressure, venous congestion and occlusion can lead to arterial insufficiency, mucosal necrosis and transmural necrosis. Left untreated, the ischemic bowel will perforate and form an abscess (or even fistulate to the skin) or necrotizing fasciitis will develop.

Patients are seen at all stages of this process. In general, the more advanced the local process, the sicker the patient is systemically. The mortality from an acute hernia varies from less than 1% in a young male patient with an incarcerated inguinal hernia, to approximately 30% in an elderly patient with a strangulated femoral hernia and comorbidity. It is important to remember that acute pain developing in an abdominal wall hernia may be caused by abdominal contents trapped within the sac but it may also be a result of peritonitis which will irritate the peritoneum of the hernial sac. Retroperitoneal collections of pus can also track along the inguinal canal and present with a tender swelling at the superficial ring. It can be very alarming to open the inguinal canal and find large volumes of pus discharging. Pus within the canal is fluctuant, unlike that in a hernia.

For patients with evidence of intestinal obstruction, the management strategy should be identical to that described for small bowel obstruction. When strangulation is suspected, broad-spectrum IV antibiotics are required. Discoloration of overlying skin is an important sign of underlying ischemia or infarction. Careful resuscitation and operative and postoperative management are especially important in elderly patients with high American Society of Anesthesiologists (ASA) grades. HDU care is ideal for ASA grades III and above (see Table 4.01).

There will be no obstruction when omentum is trapped within the hernial sac. Infarction of the omentum produces local pain and tenderness but does not produce the systemic complications associated with intestinal infarction. Other organs may be

Class I

The patient has no organic, physiological, biochemical or psychiatric disturbance. The pathological process for which surgery is to be performed is localized and does not entail a systemic disturbance. For example, a fit patient with an inguinal hernia or a fibroid uterus in an otherwise healthy woman.

Class II

Mild to moderate systemic disturbance caused either by the condition to be treated surgically or by other pathophysiological processes. For example, slightly limiting organic heart disease, mild diabetes, essential hypertension or anemia.

Class III

Severe systemic disturbance or disease from whatever cause, even though it may not be possible to define the degree of disability with finality. For example, severely limiting organic heart disease, severe diabetes with vascular complications, moderate to severe degrees of pulmonary insufficiency, angina pectoris or healed myocardial infarction.

Class IV

Severe systemic disorders that are already life-threatening and not always correctable by operation. For example, patients with organic heart disease showing marked signs of cardiac insufficiency, persistent angina or active myocarditis, advanced degrees of pulmonary, hepatic, renal or endocrine insufficiency.

Class V

The moribund patient who has little chance of survival but is submitted to operation in desperation. For example, a burst abdominal aneurysm with profound shock, major cerebral trauma with rapidly increasing intracranial pressure or massive pulmonary embolus. Most of these patients require operation as a resuscitative measure with little, if any, anesthesia.

Table 4.01 The American Society of Anesthesiologists classification of physical status.

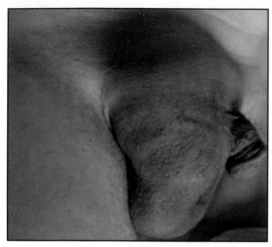

Figure 4.06 An inguinal hernia.

found within hernial sacs, but this diagnosis is rarely made preoperatively. When intestinal obstruction or strangulation is present then general anesthetic is usual. However, inguinal and femoral hernias can be repaired, and small bowel resections can be carried out under spinal or epidural anesthesia.

Inguinal hernias

Most inguinal hernias (see Figure 4.06) presenting as emergencies are relatively easy to diagnose (as long as the groin is examined). In the majority of cases the patient will present with a sudden onset of pain and swelling, and will direct the surgeon to a newly developed lump, or a lump with a recently developed irreducibility. The contents of the hernia are usually incarcerated or obstructed; strangulation is present in only 8% of cases. Therefore, it is reasonable to attempt gentle but not forcible reduction of the hernia. Almost all cases can be managed operatively through the inguinal incision alone. Any acutely irreducible and tender hernia should be operated on as soon as can be arranged. Some large femoral hernias can be difficult to distinguish from inguinal hernias; they become larger and expand upwards so that part of the hernia lies above the inguinal ligament. Their bulk and tenderness also makes location of the pubic tubercle difficult. This distinction is not critical as the true nature of the hernia is easily made at the time of surgery and the skin incision can be extended if necessary.

Femoral hernias

The margins of a femoral hernia (see Figure 4.07) are: medially the lacunar ligament, anteriorly the inguinal ligament, posteriorly the pectinal ligament, and laterally the femoral vein. The unyielding margins result in a greater risk of

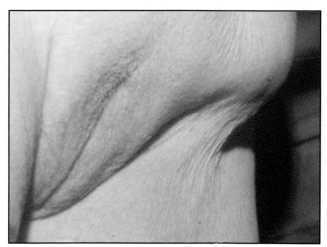

Figure 4.07 A femoral hernia.

obstruction and strangulation. Femoral hernias frequently occur in elderly patients with significant co-existing medical problems. The diagnosis must be considered in every patient presenting with intestinal obstruction. Richter's hernias (where only part of the intestinal wall is trapped within the femoral opening) are still missed because of their small size and because many elderly patients are not aware of groin tenderness or swelling. Their presence will only be detected by specific and careful examination of the femoral canal.

Surgery for femoral hernias should be straightforward and much ink has been wasted writing about the best surgical technique. It is far more important and difficult to optimize resuscitation and postoperative care. Many more patients will die of cardiorespiratory, rather than surgical complications.

Incisional hernias

Incisional hernias (see Figure 4.08) can also be irreducible, obstructed or strangulated. Even very long-standing irreducible incisional hernias can become obstructed or strangulated. The decision to operate is often delayed because of concerns about the degree of difficulty of the surgery involved and an inappropriate expectation of spontaneous resolution of the problem. The same criteria for surgery exists: any acutely irreducible tender incisional hernia should be explored and repaired.

Always look carefully at the skin at the apex of the hernia. If this is dusky or ischemic then an underlying infarcted bowel is likely. Surgery should be performed as soon as the patient can be made fit to withstand a general anesthetic.

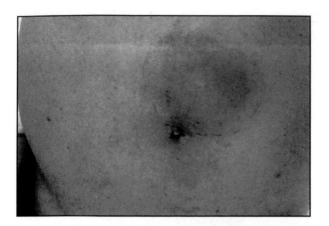

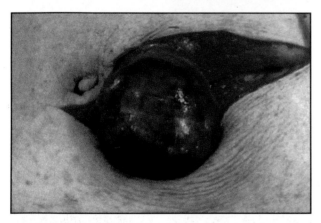

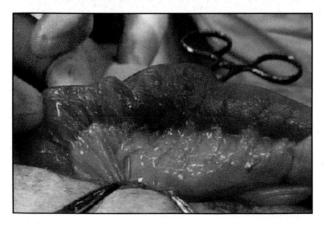

Figure 4.08 Paraumbilical hernia presenting acutely: (a) slight discoloration over the paraumbilical hernia; (b) ischemic peritoneum; and (c) surprisingly the trapped small bowel is visible.

With all types of hernia the following questions should be asked:
- are there any co-existing medical problems?
- is there any evidence of intestinal obstruction?
- how advanced is the natural history? (assess hydration)
- is there evidence of strangulation?

Investigation
- full blood count
- hematocrit
- WBC (a high count may indicate strangulation)
- U&E
- erect chest x-ray, supine abdomen
- electrocardiogram in patients over 50 years old

Management

- oxygen
- IV crystalloid, guided by the clinical degree of dehydration
- pulse monitoring
- BP monitoring
- CVP monitoring (in elderly)
- urine output
- defer surgery until you and the anesthetist are confident resuscitation has been adequate
- NG tube if there is evidence of intestinal obstruction
- a catheter can remove the bladder from the equation
- deep vein thrombosis (DVT) prophylaxis
- IV broad-spectrum antibiotics when bowel resection is necessary

Prevent the anesthetist giving the hernia a squeeze! Always identify the portion of the intestine that was trapped to see if it is viable.

Postoperative care
Expect cardiorespiratory complications in the elderly and always use the HDU in high-risk cases (ASA grade III and above).

DATE 7/11			FLUID INTAKE				FLUID OUTPUT		
INSTRUCTIONS	TIME	ORAL	Other intake				URINE	Other output	
						S/SCALE RATE	URINE	BM	
	10.00								
	11.00						Vomit + free drainage from NG		
	12.00								
	13.00								
Pump	14.00		N/Saline	300mls					
No. 43	15.00								
	16.00						50mls		Bowels
Check	17.00		5% Dextrose	200mls			600mls (Aron) Green fluid	15·2	open profuse amount
17.15	18.00		50ml N/Saline F50 Units Actrapid			4mls/hr.		15·8	
PF.	19.00					"	400mls vomit	17·8	
No. 65	20.00		N/Saline	500mls	1X2Ly	"	60mls vomit	—	
Check PF	21.00					3mls/hr.	100ml Svomit Cannula	10·2	
18.15	22.00		1unit gelofusin start 500		stopped	4ml/hr	200mls+2cmls 0	6·8	
	23.00		N/Saline	500ml	500ml/hr	1ml/hr	100mls 100+30mls 0	5·1	
	24.00	N/Saline 500	Gelofusin	500 stat	500ml/hr.	1ml/hr	150mls 250 13	5·2	
	1.00	N/Saline 500		01·30 +250	500m/h	1ml/hr.	100mls 5 18	5·2	
	2.00				250m/hr	1ml/hr	150mls		
	3.00		N/Saline 500ml		250ml/hr	1ml/hr	— 25 43	6·2	
	4.00				250Ly	1ml/hr.	—		
	5.00		0·45 N. Saline KCl 500mls		250m/hr	1ml/hr	— 30 73	7·0	
	6.00				250m/hr	1ml/hr			
	7.00		Gelofusin 500stat		250m/hr	1ml/hr	— 35 108	7·3	
	8.00		Gelofusin Stat				100 208		
	9.00		N/Saline		500ml/hr.	1ml/hr.	80ml NG 46 254	5·9	Bowels +++
SUB TOTALS							254		

DATE 8.11.99			FLUID INTAKE				FLUID OUTPUT			
INSTRUCTIONS	TIME	ORAL	Other intake				URINE HOURLY	TOTAL	Other output	
			IV Fluids	RATE	S/Scale Insulin	BM			VOMIT	NG
Pumpcheck Insulin 65. Fluids 48.8P	10.00		N/ Saline	500ml/hr	1ml/hr		40	40	—	—
	11.00		Gelofusine 'Stat'	Stat	2ml/hr	7·4	10	50	—	—
	12.00			Stat	2ml/hr		3	53	—	—
	13.00		Gelofusine	Stat.	1ml/hr.	6·6.	2	55	—	—
	14.00		Gelofusine	Stat.			35	90	—	—
	15.00									
	16.00									

Figure 4.09 Observation charts from a patient with intestinal ischemia. Hypotension, tachycardia and oliguria are not responsive to resuscitation.

Intestinal ischemia

Intestinal ischemia is rare, difficult to diagnose and highly dangerous. Obstruction of the arterial supply is more common than venous occlusion (mesenteric venous thrombosis). The small bowel mucosa is highly sensitive to ischemia. As the mucosa becomes damaged the mucosal barrier is lost and translocation of endotoxin and bacteria occurs. This ischemic environment promotes the growth of anaerobic

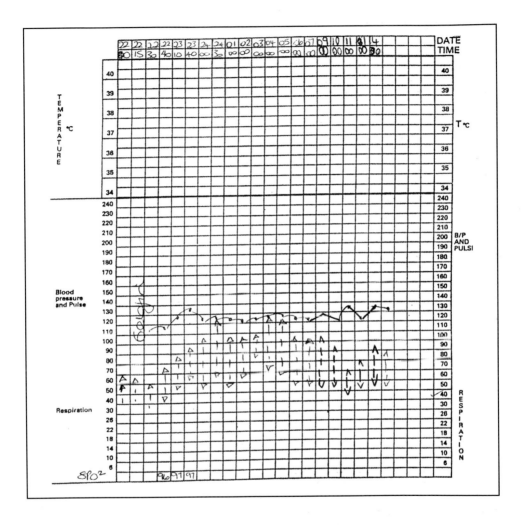

organisms, including clostridial species. For any significant length of intestinal ischemia (30 cm or greater) the patient will usually succumb to the systemic consequences of the dead bowel before perforation occurs. There is a risk of necrosis extending to adjacent tissues. If the skin overlying a hernia is deep red-purple or black, strongly suspect underlying dead tissue and arrange urgent exploration.

Presentation

Ischemia is extremely painful. The ischemic bowel causes little in the way of peritoneal irritation and the abdominal signs are limited. The classical presentation

47

of intestinal ischemia is severe abdominal pain, out of context with the degree of abdominal tenderness. Diarrhea occurs in about 50% of patients with intestinal ischemia and, when present, 80% of stool samples will be fecal occult blood positive. The presentation is also greatly influenced by the length of ischemic bowel. One of the hallmarks of mesenteric artery occlusion is profound hypotension that is unresponsive to vigorous resuscitation (see Figure 4.09).

Acute arterial occlusion may be embolic or thrombotic. The distinction is not usually of clinical importance as laparotomy is rarely performed before the ischemia is irreversible. Resection is safer than embolectomy as reperfusion of ischemic bowel carries a high risk of reperfusion injury, leading to multiple system organ injury. In addition to intraluminal vessel occlusion, infarction may result from extrinsic compression (e.g. strangulated hernia, closed loop obstruction or volvulus). In this situation too, reperfusion of the torted or obstructed bowel can be more dangerous than excision.

Suspect intestinal ischemia in any patient with abdominal pain who has co-existing cardiac disease, particularly if there is recent evidence of:

- arrhythmias (acute or chronic)
- myocardial infarction
- coronary artery bypass surgery

No biochemical test is specific for intestinal ischemia, but acidosis with increased lactate levels support the diagnosis. Most of us are aware that a high WBC count (greater than 20×10^9/L) is commonly found. A moderate increase in amylase is often detected.

Confirmation of the diagnosis is rarely made radiologically. Plain x-rays may show edema in the wall but will rarely show gas within the bowel wall. Radiology can be useful in conditions that present less acutely, such as mesenteric venous thrombosis. CT scanning may show gas within the bowel wall and thickened mucosa. Arteriography can provide direct evidence of arterial occlusion. However, even arteriography cannot exclude small areas of bowel infarction. With these other detection methods showing failings, laparotomy is necessary when there is a suspicion of ischemia.

Appendicitis

Almost all medical students are aware of the classical presentation of acute appendicitis. This develops over 1–2 days with vague central abdominal pain radiating to the right iliac fossa with associated nausea and/or vomiting (usually of short duration). Patients with appendicitis are rarely hungry. Children almost always vomit. Minor disturbances of bowel function are common and the patient is usually slightly toxic with a temperature that may reach 38–38.5°C (rarely higher) and a pulse rate of 80–120/minute. Examination reveals tenderness over McBurney's point with guarding and rebound. It has been a strict rule of surgery that a rectal examination is required in all patients with suspected acute appendicitis. This remains true in adult patients but is not always required in young children. Elaborate scoring systems have been designed to aid in the diagnosis of acute appendicitis but they are rarely used in clinical practice. Appendicitis remains a clinical diagnosis.

The WBC level is nearly always measured; it is elevated in most but not all cases of acute appendicitis. Therefore, greater reliance should be placed on the clinical assessment rather than the WBC count. Occasional patients will describe a similar attack previously.

Other presentations

Other clinical presentations depend on the position of the appendix and the progression of the illness. Dysuria is common when the inflamed appendix is in the pelvis and is pressing against the bladder or uterus. Abdominal tenderness may be absent if the appendix is entirely pelvic. Pelvic inflammation results in cervical excitation on rectal examination, and a mid-stream urine test may show an increased WBC count.

When the appendix is retro-cecal, abdominal signs tend to be less marked. Inflammation over the psoas may be detected if extension of the thigh is painful.

The natural history of acute appendicitis may be: resolution, formation of an abscess, phlegmon (appendix mass) or peritonitis. When the inflammatory process remains localized then an abscess or appendix mass results, and diagnosis is made by a combination of clinical examination and ultrasound or CT imaging. Any pus that is present should be drained. This is best achieved at open operation.

Patients with an appendix mass should be admitted, treated with bed rest, IV fluids and broad-spectrum antibiotics. They should be observed until there is good clinical evidence that the inflammation is resolving; this is usually indicated by a reduction in the pulse rate, temperature and size of the mass. Interval appendectomy is performed 6–12 weeks after discharge.

The differential diagnosis of appendix mass includes Crohn's disease and cecal carcinoma. If either of these are suspected, a barium enema is advisable prior to appendectomy.

With most diseases, the more advanced the presentation, the easier the clinical diagnosis. In appendicitis the reverse is true; diagnosis actually becomes more difficult as the disease proceeds. When patients with acute appendicitis present with or are allowed to develop generalized peritonitis, then the clinical picture changes significantly. An antecedent history in keeping with appendicitis is sometimes available. Vomiting and dehydration are common, the usual systemic signs of sepsis are present and the abdomen is typically distended secondary to paralytic ileus with generalized or lower abdominal tenderness. When acute appendicitis presents in this way, it can be indistinguishable from other causes of peritonitis with the correct diagnosis only being made at laparotomy.

Differential diagnosis

Most errors in diagnosis occur in young women, those at the extremes of life and when patients are seen in the more advanced stages of the disease. The differential diagnosis in young women includes ectopic pregnancy, torted or ruptured ovarian cyst, acute salpingitis and endometriosis. As there is an abnormal menstrual history in over 90% of patients with ectopic pregnancy, it is essential to take a history from all women of reproductive years who present as an emergency with lower abdominal pain; a pregnancy test should be performed. Patients with pelvic inflammatory disease may have a history of per vaginal discharge and have cervical excitation on per rectal examination. If an ovarian cyst ruptures or twists then the onset of pain is very sudden and gastrointestinal symptoms are less common than with acute appendicitis. The presence of rigors is atypical in appendicitis but common in acute renal and biliary infections.

In the absence of a clear clinical diagnosis of acute appendicitis, a pelvic ultrasound is often helpful for the identification of ectopic pregnancy and ovarian or endometriotic cysts. It is common to be reminded on pelvic ultrasound reports that 'an ectopic pregnancy cannot be excluded'. The combination of a negative pregnancy test and a normal pelvic ultrasound makes ectopic pregnancy extremely unlikely.

The only certain way to make an accurate diagnosis in this age group is to look directly at the potentially inflamed organs. There is good evidence to support the use of diagnostic laparoscopy for this purpose. However, laparoscopy is not always available, particularly after 5 pm, and the diagnostic decision is therefore 'is the patient sufficiently unwell to merit a general anesthetic and a right iliac fossa muscle splitting incision'. In the early stages of appendicitis a wait-and-see policy is safe as long as ectopic pregnancy has been excluded and the patient is regularly reviewed. A lower threshold for appendectomy has been accepted for young women because of concerns about infertility associated with pelvic sepsis. A recent large study from Scandinavia has provided good evidence that the risk of infertility following appendicitis is not increased and that the threshold for appendectomy should be the same for all females of reproductive years.

There is no generally accepted rate for removing normal appendixes, although a figure of 30% is often quoted. The senior house officer should keep a record of these cases to know what the diagnostic accuracy rate is.

Postoperative care

- Day 1—oral intake increased to free fluids
- Day 2—diet introduced if fluids are tolerated
- Home when eating and drinking, bowels open, apyrexial and mobile

Postoperative antibiotics are given by most surgeons:

- if the appendix is non-perforated, 500 mg of Flagyl should be administered rectally or IV at 8 and 16 hours after the operation
- if the appendix is perforated administer broad-spectrum IV antibiotics for 48 hours
- administer DVT prophylaxis if the patient is obese, taking the oral contraceptive pill or has pelvic sepsis

chapter 5

Large bowel problems
Ian MacLennan & James Hill

Large bowel obstruction

The cardinal features of large and small bowel obstruction are the same:

- colicky abdominal pain
- vomiting
- absolute constipation
- abdominal distension

With large bowel obstruction, in contrast to obstruction of the small bowel, distension occurs early and vomiting later. The distal unobstructed colon is emptied by normal peristalsis and the colon above the obstruction distends with gas and semi-solid feces as far as the ileo-cecal valve. If the valve is incompetent, this decompresses the colon and the risk of perforation is greatly decreased. If the ileo-cecal valve is competent, there is a closed loop obstruction and the colon continues to dilate. The cecum is capable of the greatest distension and is the part of the colon in most danger of perforation. When the cecal diameter is greater than 14 cm, the risk of perforation is much greater. Localized tenderness over the cecum and right iliac fossa peritonism should also raise concerns.

Presentation
Patients with an obstructing cancer often give no previous history suggestive of colonic carcinoma, i.e. change in bowel habit or rectal bleeding. On examination the distended colon is sometimes discernible, but it is more common simply to encounter a distended abdomen with obstructed bowel sounds. It is uncommon to find a mass on abdominal examination. Rectal examination is mandatory, but it is unusual to find a low rectal cancer presenting with obstruction because of the diameter of the rectal ampulla. A sigmoid carcinoma in the pouch of Douglas is sometimes palpable through the rectal wall. A ballooned rectum is suggestive of pseudo-obstruction.

53

Investigation

Investigations include a full blood count, urea and electrolytes, group and save, an erect chest x-ray and a supine abdominal x-ray. On plain abdominal x-ray the following questions should be asked:

(a) are the findings suggestive of large bowel obstruction?

(b) what is the cecal diameter?

If the x-ray shows a dilated colon, with or without small bowel dilatation, the answer to question (a) is yes (see Figure 5.01).

> **!** Mechanical large bowel obstruction cannot be diagnosed on a plain abdominal x-ray.

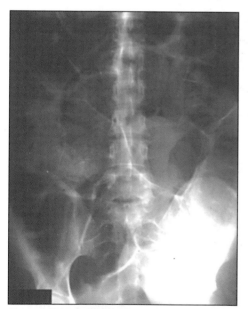

Figure 5.01 Mechanical large bowel obstruction.

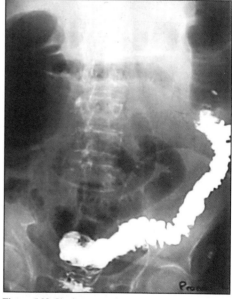

Figure 5.02 Single contrast barium enema confirming mechanical obstruction.

However experienced you are, colonic pseudo-obstruction is indistinguishable from mechanical obstruction. A single contrast enema is the investigation of choice for this patient (see Figure 5.02).

> **!** Do not give Picolax or any other bowel preparation before the barium enema as these may cause rupture of the obstructed colon.

The urgency of the investigation is based on the likelihood of colonic perforation. Thus, if the abdomen is soft with no cecal tenderness and the cecal diameter is below 14 cm, it should be safe to carry out the investigation within 24 hours. If the cecum is tender or over 14 cm in diameter, the x-ray should be performed as soon as practically possible. The surgical resident should try to observe the contrast enema being performed. The radiologist sometimes needs encouragement to persist in an elderly patient who is struggling to hold onto the barium. It is also helpful to look at the plain x-rays with the radiologist for educational purposes.

Management

- oxygen
- rehydration (as for small bowel obstruction)
- analgesia and anti-emetics
- nasogastric tube insertion
- consent
- laparotomy

Obtaining consent should include an explanation of the necessity for surgery. Say that this is a major operation carried out as an emergency procedure and therefore carries a significant risk. You should say that without an operation the patient will not survive. If you find it helpful to discuss chances of survival, a mortality rate of 20% is found in most series. High dependency unit (HDU) or intensive care unit (ICU) nursing may be required. It is essential to warn the patient that a stoma may be necessary and that it may be permanent. Get the stoma therapist to site the stoma.

Volvulus

A colonic volvulus arises when a mobile loop of colon twists around a narrow mesentery. Complications arise from obstruction of the lumen of the bowel and ischemia if the torsion occludes the blood supply. Presentation is similar to other causes of large bowel obstruction.

Sigmoid volvulus is much more common than cecal volvulus and easier to diagnose. In patients with sigmoid volvulus, the distended sigmoid colon is sometimes discernible through the abdominal wall. The diagnosis is confirmed on plain abdominal x-ray. If you are in doubt, discuss the x-ray with senior staff. Management is within the capabilities of the surgical resident. Decompression is safe as long as there is no clinical evidence of sigmoid colon ischemia (soft abdomen with no peritonism and a normal white blood cell [WBC] count). Cecal and sigmoid volvulus are compared in Table 5.01.

	Cecal	Sigmoid
Age	30–40	Over 70
Male to female ratio	1:3	3:1
Predisposing factors	None known	Longstanding constipation Anticholinergic drugs
Diagnosis	Rarely made preoperatively	Diagnosis readily made
Treatment	Right hemicolectomy	Endoscopic decompression +/- surgical resection
Prognosis	Good	High morbidity and mortality

Table 5.01 Cecal and sigmoid volvulus compared.

Equipment required

• rigid sigmoidoscope
• well lubricated flatus tube (gastric lavage tube if the former is unavailable)
• gloves and aprons (wet suit and goggles)
• incontinence pads
• bucket

The first time you attempt to deflate a volvulus make sure you have someone with you who has previous experience. The rigid sigmoidoscope is introduced into the upper rectum. Make sure that the sigmoidoscope is in the lumen and not pushed hard against the rectal wall. The lubricated tube is then pushed gently through the sigmoidoscope and into the dilated colon. Deflation is usually instant and obvious. Further decompression can be achieved by pressing on the abdominal wall. Leave the tube *in situ* for around 24 hours until a repeat plain x-ray confirms decompression (see Figure 5.03).

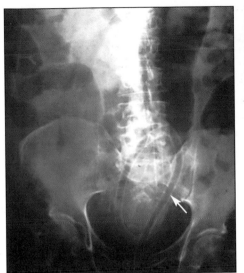 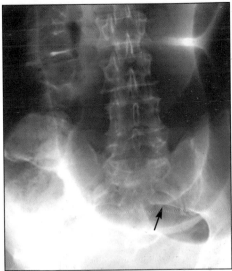

Figure 5.03 Sigmoid volvulus following decompression with a flatus tube *in situ* (arrow).

Figure 5.04 Sigmoid volvulus (arrow).

When is laparotomy required?

- when initial decompression is unsuccessful

- when volvulus is recurrent – this occurs in up to 50% of cases, and where possible laparotomy is delayed until colonic edema has settled; this may take a few days

- when there is evidence of colonic ischemia

The x-ray appearances of sigmoid and cecal volvulus are shown (see Figures 5.04 and 5.05).

Colonic pseudo-obstruction

More than 100 causes of pseudo-obstruction have been described; there is no benefit to be gained from learning all of these. The most common causes are fluid and electrolyte disturbances, renal failure and sepsis.

It is important to appreciate that the diagnosis is one of exclusion, having performed a single contrast gastrografin or dilute barium enema. If the patient is passing loose stools in association with colonic distension, then acute colitis, pseudo-membranous colitis in particular, should be excluded by sending a stool sample for *Clostridium difficile* analysis.

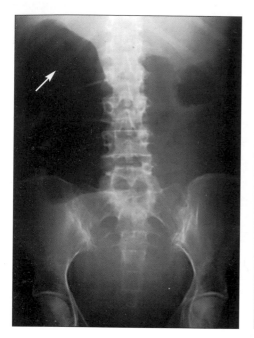

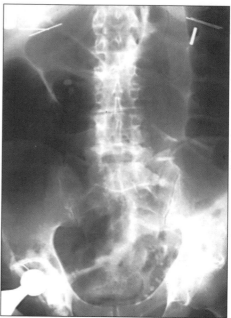

Figure 5.05 Cecal volvulus, note that it is more common to make the diagnosis at laparotomy than on the basis of the plain abdominal x-ray (arrow).

Figure 5.06 Colonic pseudo-obstruction; this cannot be distinguished from mechanical large bowel obstruction (see Figure 5.01). The cecum is grossly distended (16 cm diameter) and edematous and in imminent danger of rupture.

Disaster scenario one

A 75-year-old man presents with classic features of large bowel obstruction. Investigations reveal elevated potassium and urea. A plain abdominal x-ray shows a grossly dilated colon to recto-sigmoid (see Figure 5.06). The patient is resuscitated and a laparotomy performed. No obstructing lesion is found and a diagnosis of pseudo-obstruction, secondary to renal failure, is made. The patient is transferred to HDU but, despite appropriate treatment, he deteriorates and dies of cardiorespiratory complications 4 days after the operation. The coroner writes to you and asks for a report! This simple case reminds us that all patients with suspected mechanical large bowel obstruction need single contrast enemas.

Perforation can occur with pseudo-obstruction. As with mechanical obstruction, the cecum is most likely to rupture so look particularly for tenderness over the cecum and a diameter of over 14 cm. If these features are present, decompression is urgently required. Decompression can be achieved pharmacologically with 2 mg of intravenous (IV) neostigmine with cardiac monitoring because of the risk of bradycardia. If neostigmine fails, colonoscopic decompression can be attempted. Subtotal colectomy is performed if there is impending or actual cecal rupture despite conservative treatment.

Diverticulitis

Acute diverticulitis is caused by an acute infection occurring in and around a diverticulum. The sigmoid colon is almost always involved.

There are four possible outcomes for a patient with diverticulitis:

- **resolution** if the infection is localized or low-grade
- **abscess** which can vary in size from a small pericolic collection to a large abscess extending into the pelvis
- **perforation** with the inflammatory process producing a free perforation in the colon which results in generalized peritonitis; alternatively an abscess may rupture also causing generalized peritonitis
- **phlegmon** with the acute infection or inflammation extending to adjacent organs causing them to become matted together without an abscess forming

On admission, patients with localized or low-grade infection, and those with a free perforation, are relatively easy to differentiate. The patient with low-grade localized sepsis presents with the so called 'left-sided appendicitis'. The history is of pain in the left iliac fossa associated with minor degrees of bowel disturbance, either constipation or loose stools. The patient with localized sepsis is systemically well with a mild tachycardia and pyrexia. Examination reveals localized tenderness, rebound and guarding. Rectal examination reveals at most some left-sided tenderness.

The patient with generalized peritonitis, secondary to diverticular perforation, is in severe pain. Constipation is usual and vomiting may be present due to pain and intestinal paralysis. On examination the patient looks generally unwell, has a tachycardia and is often hypotensive (note that in elderly patients a blood pressure [BP] of 120/80 mmHg may be significantly lower than normal). The abdomen is distended and abdominal tenderness is widespread with rebound. The board-like rigidity seen in perforated peptic ulcer disease is often absent, especially in elderly patients. The presence or absence of bowel sounds is not diagnostic; it is more common to hear a few high pitched bowel sounds or nothing. A plain abdominal x-ray showing a large amount of free gas is very suggestive of colonic perforation (see Figure 5.07).

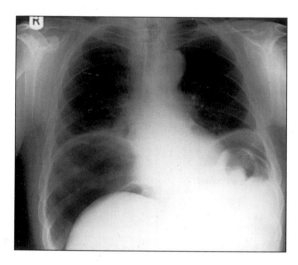

Figure 5.07 Suspect colonic perforation when there is a large volume of free intraperitoneal gas.

The patient with localized or low-grade sepsis should recover within 48–72 hours if treated appropriately with IV fluid, resting the gastrointestinal (GI) tract and broad-spectrum IV antibiotics.

The patient with generalized peritonitis will require aggressive resuscitation in the HDU or ICU with central monitoring, followed by laparotomy. Postoperative HDU or ICU care is appropriate as systemic inflammatory response syndrome is common and a mortality rate of 25% can be expected.

The patient with neither localized left iliac fossa signs nor generalized peritonitis is more difficult to assess and predict an outcome. A typical patient in this group has lower abdominal peritonism, mild distension, scanty bowel sounds, a tachycardia of 90–110/minute, is normotensive and has a temperature of around 38°C. This patient's sepsis could resolve or progress and there is no method for determining this other than regular review of the patient. On review every 3–4 hours, take note of the pain and analgesic requirements, any change in abdominal signs, pulse, respiratory rate, BP and urine output. Any evidence of spreading peritonitis or worsening systemic sepsis with falling BP and urine output, despite appropriate treatment, should be managed by laparotomy.

Another common scenario is the patient who is not improving as expected 48 hours after treatment. Neither the sepsis has resolved nor has the patient developed generalized peritonitis. The single most informative investigation under these circumstances is an abdominal computed tomography (CT) scan with contrast to look for an abscess and any evidence of perforation. The radiologist may prefer to give the contrast orally but there is evidence of increased accuracy if the contrast is given rectally. Where possible, emergency laparotomy should be avoided as it carries such a high morbidity and mortality and usually results in stoma formation. The aim is to 'downstage' the disease to increase the chances of resolution without surgery or to produce a less septic patient if surgery is ultimately required. Abscesses can be drained percutaneously or transrectally and the drain left *in situ* until the collection has resolved. Confirmation of resolution can be demonstrated clinically by ultrasound or a repeat CT scan, depending on the complexity of the abscess.

Other investigations

- sigmoidoscopy is rarely indicated, it will not provide any information about the extra-colonic inflammation and is potentially dangerous
- barium enema examination is indicated when the acute inflammation has resolved to confirm the diagnosis and exclude mucosal disease
- ultrasound scanning can be useful in the absence of CT but it is less accurate for the diagnosis of a pelvic abscess or a small collection in a large area of inflammation

Conservative therapy (regular review)	Surgical therapy
Localized signs	Diffuse peritonitis
No free gas	Free gas
Patient systemically well	Patient hypotensive and hypoxic

Table 5.02 Conservative versus surgical therapy for the treatment of diverticulitis.

Lower gastrointestinal bleeding

To determine the blood loss ask the following questions:
- what is the estimated total volume of blood loss?
- has the patient collapsed or lost consciousness as a result of the bleeding?
- are there compensatory effects of bleeding on the cardiorespiratory system?

Description of the color of the blood can be useful, but avoid at all costs the description 'fresh malena'. In general, blood from the stomach, duodenum and proximal small bowel will be black and blood from the left colon bright or dark red. Be aware that very brisk upper

GI bleeding can be red. Always perform a rectal examination and study the blood on the examining finger. Blood is an effective purgative and if the patient is bleeding actively the blood will be passed rectally. It is unusual to find large volumes of retained blood in the colon. With the combination of the description of the blood, the urea/creatinine ratio and lack of symptoms or predisposing factors for peptic ulcer disease, it is possible to differentiate upper and lower GI bleeding in almost all cases. (See Table 5.03).

	Upper GI bleeding	**Lower GI bleeding**
Hematemesis	May be present	Absent
Color of stool	Black	Dark/bright red
Urea/creatinine ratio	>100	<100
Risk factors	Non-steroidal drugs	
	Steroids	
	Previous peptic ulcer	
	Symptoms of peptic ulcer	

Table 5.03 Characteristics of upper and lower GI bleeding compared.

By definition, lower GI bleeding is from a site beyond the D-J flexure (see Figure 5.08). Lower GI bleeding will resolve spontaneously in 90% of cases. Angiodysplasia (see Figure 5.09) is the most common cause of lower GI bleeding followed by diverticular disease; bleeding is more common in the elderly and in patients with aortic valve disease, especially if they are anticoagulated. Life-threatening bleeding from tumors or inflammatory bowel disease is rare.

It is important to be aware of potentially life-threatening bleeding from pathology close to the anal canal. This includes rectal varices (see Figure 5.10), hemorrhoids and a solitary rectal ulcer. Rectal or anal canal causes of lower GI bleeding typically present with recurrent (every 20–30 minutes) passage of 50–200 mL of blood that appears fresh and contains clots. This is similar to the presentation of postoperative bleeding after hemorrhoidectomy. For these patients, urgent examination under anesthesia (EUA) and sigmoidoscopy are indicated.

Investigation
- FBC
- urea/creatine ratio less than 100
- cross-match (at least 2 units but judge this on estimated blood loss and rate of blood loss)
- clotting screen

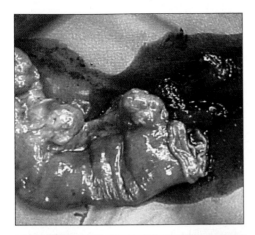

Figure 5.08 Jejunal diverticulosis. Bleeding beyond the D–J flexure is lower GI bleeding.

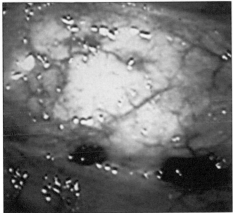

Figure 5.09 Angiodysplasia. This is the most common cause of lower GI bleeding.

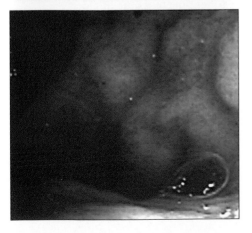

Figure 5.10 Rectal varices. It is important to remember that torrential GI hemorrhage can occur from the rectum and anal canal.

Management

> - nil by mouth
> - IV injection with crystalloid, colloid or blood to maintain BP and a urine output of 30–50 mL/hour
> - transfuse to achieve hemoglobin (Hb) of approximately 10 g/dL

Patients at greater risk of requiring surgical intervention are those with large estimated losses who continue to bleed and those who have frequent episodes of blood loss.

> **!** There is a reduced risk of spontaneous resolution if a 6-unit transfusion is required.

If the bleeding settles spontaneously it is necessary to exclude a mucosal abnormality. If the bleeding is mild and settles quickly this can be safely done on an out-patient basis, either by colonoscopy or barium enema. For more severe bleeding it is reassuring to investigate as an in-patient. It is uncommon to find a specific cause for the bleeding. If mucosal disease can be excluded, additional investigations are not required as further bleeding is rare. Further investigations are required if the bleeding does not stop. Definitive investigations are more likely to be positive if the patient is actively bleeding. It is recommended that all patients have an upper GI endoscopy to exclude an upper GI cause for the bleeding. Attempts to find the site or segment of colon that is bleeding are important as blind hemicolectomy carries too great a risk of not excising the bleeding site. The risk is reduced with total colectomy but this is a major procedure and is associated with a poor functional outcome in elderly patients.

Several techniques can be used for investigation

Colonoscopy – some surgeons have described high success rates in identifying the bleeding site using this technique. When the site of bleeding is detected it can be stopped endoscopically by injection with dilute adrenaline or with argon beam plasma coagulation. If there is a large volume of blood in the colon, it is the limit of most surgeon's expectations to pass the colonoscope to the splenic flexure. Thus, if blood is seen proximal to the splenic flexure then the right colon is the most likely source of the blood and extended right hemicolectomy (to the splenic flexure) is the most likely procedure to be required. Colonic bleeding does not travel a significant distance proximally but anorectal bleeding can pass retrogradely into the left colon, much like an enema.

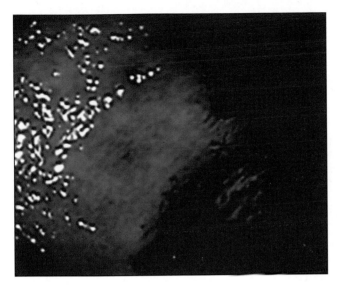

Figure 5.11 Coating of the colonic mucosa with blood makes identification of small bleeding lesions such as angiodysplasia difficult.

Arteriography – active bleeding at a rate of 0.5 mL/minute is required for the bleeding point to be detectable. To perform the examination while the patient is actively bleeding requires a 24-hour angiography service which is not available in all centers. Even if the bleeding appears to have stopped, angiography may be useful for identifying angiodysplasia. Surgical excision will be guided if an active bleeding point can be identified but it is more useful if the feeding vessel can be occluded radiologically. The success rate of radiological intervention is high and the risk of infarction, perforation and stricture is small.

Red cell labeling – red cells are removed, radiolabeled, reinjected and the abdomen is scanned with a gamma camera to look for pooling of radioactivity at the site of bleeding. Whilst good success rates are claimed, it is used less frequently than the other two techniques and is not therapeutic.

Other useful investigations when the source of bleeding remains obscure include a CT scan with oral contrast and small bowel contrast studies. These tests will identify small bowel lesions. There is evidence to support the use of laparotomy for patients who continue to bleed in the presence of normal investigations. Intraoperative colonoscopy is performed at the time of laparotomy when the colon can be cleaned by irrigation fluid introduced via the appendix. This technique increases the likelihood of identifying the bleeding site and guides surgical resection more accurately.

Disaster scenario two

A fit 66-year-old man is admitted with a large, dark red rectal bleed. The estimated volume of blood loss is 1 L and there is no previous history or other symptoms.

Examination
- pulse 120/minute
- BP 90/60 mmHg
- the abdomen is soft and on per rectal (PR) examination dark red blood is seen on the glove
- Hb 6.3 g/dL
- urea 6.5 mmol/L
- creatinine 0.089 mmol/L (urea/creatinine ratio less than 100)
- clotting studies normal
- rigid sigmoidoscopy reveals dark red blood (++), no mucosa is seen

Acute bleeding and hypotension continues despite colloid and blood transfusion. Approximately 200 mL of blood passes every 30 minutes. The patient is urgently taken to theater. An upper GI endoscopy is normal. Intraoperative colonoscopy without lavage shows blood (+++) in the left colon and a left hemicolectomy is performed.

Further profound dark red bleeding is observed PR, 24 hours postoperatively. The patient is tachycardic, hypotensive and has a Hb level of 6.3 g/dL after a total of 12 units have been transfused. Further colonoscopy reveals blood (+++) in the colon. A second laparotomy results in complete colectomy with ileo-rectal anastomosis.

The patient develops an anastomostic leak, peritonitis and multiple system organ failure (MSOF) 6 days postoperatively. Further laparotomy with formation of an ileostomy and oversewing of the rectal stump is performed.

After 3 weeks in the ICU the patient recovers and returns to the ward. He has a further large lower GI hemorrhage 3 days later. EUA reveals a bleeding hemorrhoid (the source of the bleeding all along) and this is treated with a single transfixion suture.

Comment

The volume of blood loss and persistence of hypotension clearly indicate that intervention was required. In this case, no arteriography was available, the patient was taken to theater appropriately but no on-table colonic lavage was performed. The colectomy was therefore blind. A distal cause for hemorrhage such as hemorrhoids, rectal varices or a solitary rectal ulcer was not considered or specifically looked for. The patient had two unnecessary laparotomies and experienced the life-threatening complication of surgery.

Acute colitis

Acute colitis is encountered in patients with ulcerative colitis, Crohn's disease, indeterminate colitis and infective colitis (particularly pseudo-membranous colitis secondary to *Clostridium difficile* infection). Mucosal inflammation and ulceration result in blood and mucus loss from the rectum. The inflamed colon is painful and tender. The greater the inflammation, the greater the symptoms of bloody diarrhea, pain and tenderness. If severe enough the inflammation causes systemic illness with changes in the temperature and pulse rate. Blood loss in the stool causes anemia. The inflammation and protein loss in the stool lead to low albumin levels and the mediators of the inflammation cause a pyrexia and leukocytosis. As most of these factors are directly related to the surface area of inflamed colon, severe colitis with systemic changes is much more common in total or near total colitis compared to segmental colitis.

The severity of the inflammation is also correlated with the likelihood of requiring urgent colectomy. The most severe forms of inflammation result in toxic dilatation or disintegrative colitis. The etiology of toxic dilatation is poorly understood. When it occurs, the colon (particularly the transverse colon) is dilated and peristaltic activity is lost. The colonic wall becomes thin and weak and perforates easily. In disintegrative colitis the wall is equally weak and thin and susceptible to perforation but not acutely dilated. The key is to recognize when the patient is at high risk of colonic perforation. Morbidity and mortality rise very significantly if surgery is performed after the colon has perforated. Standard treatment for acute colitis is in-patient care with high-dose IV steroids (commonly hydrocortisone at 100 mg qds), IV fluids, analgesia with or without IV antibiotics.

Within 5 days significant improvement should be seen in the following parameters:

- stool frequency
- temperature
- tachycardia
- leukocytosis
- anemia
- albumin

The on-call surgical team is usually faced with three types of patient

1 A systemically well patient improving on treatment – the surgical resident should see the patient, confirm that there is symptomatic improvement, look at the pulse and temperature chart, check the blood parameters and review regularly until discharge. It is safe to review this type of patient every 1–2 days.

2 A systemically unwell patient who is deteriorating despite maximal medical therapy – as the colon becomes diseased, it is less able to maintain peristalsis and the stool frequency reduces. This is a serious warning sign of impending perforation. This patient typically has a distended, generally tender abdomen, maximal over the colon, with worsening parameters. The plain abdominal x-ray may show signs of toxic dilatation (see Figure 5.12), but in cases of disintegrative colitis only edema is observed in the colonic wall. If the x-ray shows free gas then the decision to operate has been delayed for too long. Standard surgery is total colectomy with ileostomy and either oversewing the rectal stump or fashioning a mucus fistula.

3 A patient who is neither truly improving nor obviously deteriorating – typically some of the parameters listed above are improving or stable whilst others are deteriorating (most commonly the serum albumin). The patient has typically had 5 days of IV steroid therapy and, having converted to oral steroids, abdominal pain, stool frequency, blood and mucus slowly deteriorate again. There may be a temptation to try other, newer immunomodulators or heparin. These patients are often young and very reluctant to lose the colon and accept an ileostomy. Communication with the patient is therefore vital and should include a discussion of the possibility of surgery early on, soon after admission. Keep patients and relatives regularly updated. Showing relatives the results of investigations can often be helpful, as can involving the nursing staff and stoma therapist. The patient should be reviewed at least once daily. The need for colectomy usually becomes clearer within the following 2–3 days.

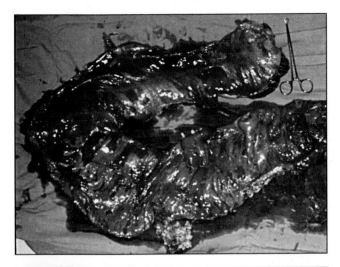

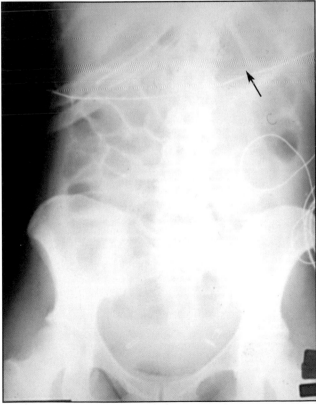

Figure 5.12 Toxic dilatation in a patient with severe pseudo-membranous colitis (arrow).

Disaster scenario three

A 26-year-old woman is admitted with colicky abdominal pain and bloody diarrhea (x10/day). She has no previous history and has recently traveled to Europe.

Examination
- temperature 38.2°C
- pulse 100/minute
- BP 100/70 mmHg
- dehydrated (+)
- abdomen slightly distended, generally tender (+), no guarding
- normal bowel sounds

Investigation
- WBC count 14.4x10^9/L
- Hb 10.3 g/dL
- platelets 535/mm^3
- albumin 30 g/L
- plain x-ray reveals mucosal edema in the left colon
- flexible sigmoidoscopy to 20 cm shows severe proctosigmoiditis, biopsy taken
- stool culture negative

Management

Day 1   Rehydration with IV crystalloid

IV hydrocortisone (100 mg qds) and rectal steroid enemas, oral 5-ASA treatment

IV cefuroxime and metronidazole

Day 2   Bowel opening (BO) x10/day, blood and mucus. Less abdominal pain

Temp 38.3°C, pulse 90/minute, normotensive

No abdominal distension, tenderness in status quo (ISQ)

WBC 11.8x10^9/L, Hb 9.6 g/dL, platelets 555/mm^3

Albumin 28 g/dL

Day 3   BOx8. Less abdominal pain, tenderness ISQ
         Temperature pulse and BP unchanged
         FBC unchanged
         Albumin 26 g/dL

Day 4   BOx7. Pain and tenderness unchanged
         Temperature 38.1°C, pulse 100/minute, normotensive
         WBC 14.4×10^9/L, Hb 9.2 g/dL
         Albumin 26 g/dL

Day 5   BOx5. Pain and tenderness unchanged
         Temperature 38.3°C, pulse 110/minute
         WBC 16×10^9/L, Hb 9.2 g/dL
         Albumin 25 g/dL

Day 6   BOx5. Pain and tenderness slightly increased
         Temperature 38.2°C, pulse 100/minute
         WBC 14.6×10^9/L, Hb 8.8 g/dL
         Albumin 25 g/dL

Day 7   BOx2. Nausea, abdominal distension, tenderness slightly increased
         again
         Temperature 38.4°C, pulse 120/minute
         WBC 17.5×10^9/L, Hb 7.6 g/dL
         Albumin 23 g/dL

Day 8   No bowel opening or flatus passed; abdominal distension increased,
         generalized tenderness (++), absent bowel sounds
         Temp 38.5°C, pulse 130/minute
         WBC 21×10^9/L, Hb 7.3 g/dL
         Laparotomy
         Perforated transverse colon, generalized peritoneal contamination
         Total colectomy with ileostomy and mucus fistula
         Patient develops MSOF, is ventilated in the ICU and requires
         hemofiltration before ultimately recovering

Comment

The patient has never really shown any significant improvement on full medical treatment after 5–6 days. At this point colectomy was the correct management. Failure to progress is just as important as deterioration. It is psychologically more difficult for the surgeon to operate when the patient is reasonably well than when the operation is clearly life-saving. Joint management between surgeons and physicians is helpful in making decisions about the timing of surgery. Continuity of care, with the same people reviewing the patient each day, also allows easier decision making.

Ischemic colitis

The colon in the region of the splenic flexure and upper descending colon is most susceptible to ischemia. The etiology is uncertain in most patients, but it is more common in elderly patients and those with pre-existing arterial disease. The colonic mucosa is the layer of the bowel wall most sensitive to ischemia. Mucosal ischemia causes ulceration and bleeding (see Figure 5.13). If the ischemia is sufficient to cause mucosal necrosis only, the ulceration should resolve spontaneously. If it is more severe, the muscularis propria is affected. The result is either stricture formation or full thickness perforation.

Ischemic colitis is also seen after aortic surgery. The inferior mesenteric artery is temporarily or permanently occluded during this operation, and minor degrees of left colonic ischemia are common. However, full thickness ischemia of the left colonic wall is only seen after approximately 1% of aortic reconstructions (see Figure 5.14).

The ischemia causes abdominal pain. Pain is sudden in onset, moderately severe and is experienced on the left side. The blood lost from the ulcerated mucosa is dark or bright red, usually mixed with stool, and may be accompanied by mucus. The bleeding is low volume and almost never life-threatening. After the first show of blood, macroscopic bleeding usually settles. On examination the patient has a mild pyrexia and tachycardia, without significant hypotension. Tenderness is maximal over the ischemic colon with local rebound and guarding. The presence of generalized peritonitis should alert you to a different diagnosis of perforation of the ischemic colon. Free perforation is surprisingly rare. The low risk of perforation is illustrated by the fact that patients with severe colonic bleeding, secondary to angiodysplasia or diverticular disease seen on arteriography, can be treated by insertion of coils into the main feeding artery to this part of the colon; perforation and stricture following this are rare.

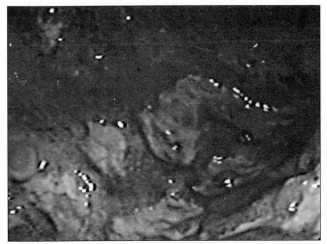

Figure 5.13 Mucosal ulceration in ischemic colitis.

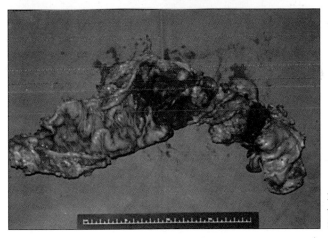

Figure 5.14 Left colonic ischemia with full thickness perforation following aortic surgery.

Investigations should reveal an elevated WBC count, and a plain x-ray should show mucosal edema (thumb printing) in the left colon (see Figure 5.15). Surgical residents are often skeptical about their ability to recognize mucosal edema, but it does occur and if you remember the appearance on the x-rays shown you will be able to recognize it (see Figure 5.16).

The most common mistaken diagnosis is diverticular disease. Acute diverticulitis is not associated with bleeding and when colonic bleeding is secondary to diverticular disease there are no significant signs of inflammation.

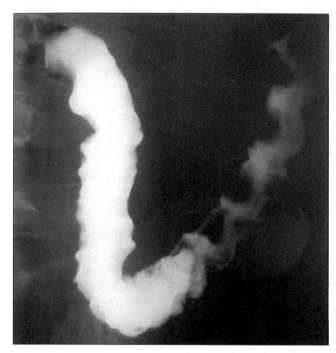

Figure 5.15 Left colonic mucosal edema with thumb printing in a patient with ischemic colitis.

Management

- IV crystalloid
- IV antibiotics to cover colonic organisms
- resting of the GI tract

Outcomes in order of frequency are: resolution, stricture formation and perforation. Conservative measures are employed in the absence of generalized peritonitis. Improvement is associated with reduction in abdominal pain and tenderness, restoration of bowel function and a falling WBC count. At some point a barium enema is necessary. If performed early in the natural history of the disease, mucosal edema and luminal narrowing are common. Even when the luminal narrowing appears impressive, in many cases it will improve over time. Do not rush into operating on these patients, who are often elderly with significant comorbidity. If there is evidence of deterioration and development of peritonitis, laparotomy with resection of the ischemic colon and exteriorization or anastomosis is performed. Total colonic ischemia is rarely encountered. It is seen following coronary artery bypass surgery (see Figure 5.17).

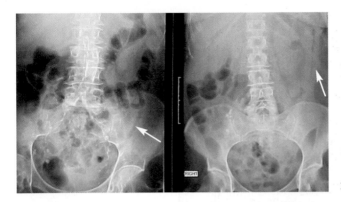

Figure 5.16 Mucosal edema (arrows).

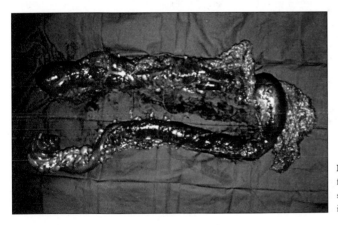

Figure 5.17 Total colonic ischemia following coronary artery bypass surgery. Left untreated, the ischemia is fatal long before perforation occurs.

Perianal sepsis

The diagnosis and treatment of perianal sepsis is often left entirely to the surgical resident.

Some simple rules must be observed:

- do not treat complex abscesses without supervision. Complex abscesses are more common in patients with a previous history of perianal sepsis, Crohn's disease, and those who have immune suppression such as human immunodeficiency virus infection
- always think about the possibility of synergistic gangrene/necrotizing fasciitis/Fournier's gangrene
- do not treat any fistula other than an obvious subcutaneous fistula

Errors commonly made by surgical residents

1 Failure to diagnose an intersphincteric abscess. The classical presentation is the patient who attends the accident and emergency department complaining of severe throbbing anal pain. On examination there is no visible abnormality but rectal examination is not possible because of pain. The patient is thought to have an acute fissure or an early abscess and is discharged with analgesia and antibiotics, only to return 24–48 hours later with unrelieved symptoms and a more complex abscess. Other perianal problems that present acutely such as a thrombosed external hemorrhoid, a thrombosed internal hemorrhoid or an acute fissure-in-ano will have a visible abnormality at the anal margin. Therefore, in the absence of any definite finding to explain the patient's symptoms, those presenting with acute severe anal pain (especially where it is not possible to perform a rectal examination) should be admitted for examination under anesthetic

2 Failure to establish adequate drainage at the time of surgery

3 Failure to guide the patient expeditiously through the theater hurdles

Management

- almost all perianal abscesses should be drained under general anesthesia. If the abscess is thought to be complex ask for senior help
- perform rigid sigmoidoscopy to look for co-existing proctitis
- palpate the anal canal carefully for an internal opening. Press on the abscess to see if any pus is visible in the anal canal. Shave the perianal skin in the region of the abscess. This makes subsequent dressing changes much easier
- send pus for culture and sensitivity. An abscess growing non-gut organisms is only rarely associated with a fistula and, therefore, should heal reliably after incision and drainage. If there is synergistic gangrene, antibiotic sensitivities are crucial
- if you suspect Crohn's disease (multiple previous abscesses or complex fistula) or malignancy send skin for histological analysis
- if you are unsure about where to make an incision, try aspirating pus with a white needle connected to a 20 cc syringe. Excise a disc of skin after making a cruciate incision sufficient to drain the abscess. Gently break down any loculi digitally but avoid aggressive probing. If the patient is found to have an unexpected complex abscess ask for senior advice. Avoid sphincter division

The stages in the treatment of a perianal abscess are demonstrated in Figure 5.18.

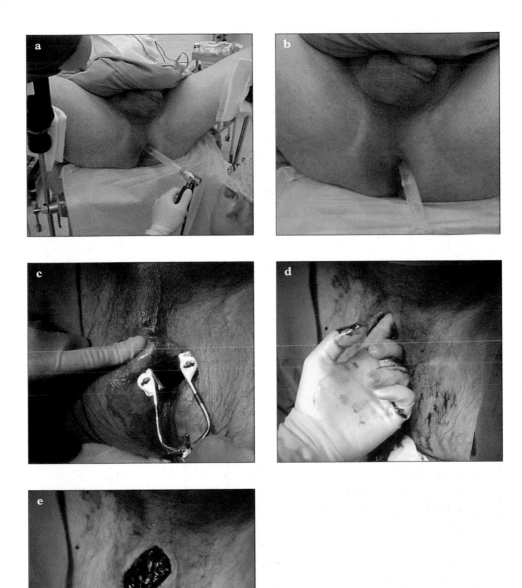

Figure 5.18 Stages in the treatment of a perianal abscess: (a) rigid sigmoidoscopy; (b) look for the site of maximal erythema and fluctuance; (c) look for an internal opening; (d) gently break down loculi digitally; (e) adequate deroofing to allow drainage.

Good News	Bad News
Small abscess	Large abscess, bilateral abscess
First abscess	Previous abscess
Young	Old
Healthy	Co-existing cardiorespiratory or renal disease
	Known Crohn's disease
	Fat
	Obese

Table 5.04 Expected outcomes for patients with perianal sepsis.

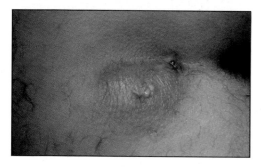

Figure 5.19 A pilonidal abscess.

Pilonidal abscess

Pilonidal abscesses are easily recognized swellings in the natal cleft (see Figure 5.19). Look carefully for midline pits and lateral tracks. A rectal examination should always be performed to exclude a perianal abscess with posterior extension towards the natal cleft. Drainage under general anesthetic is required. The patient can be placed in the left lateral position (the prone position is not required). Shave the affected area. A simple linear incision does not provide adequate drainage and will not excise the underlying pilonidal sinus. An elliptical excision is made and the sinus is excised. If you are unsure how wide the excision should be, ask. Careful hemostasis is required as persistent bleeding from the wound edge can necessitate a return to theater. Packing with ribbon gauze of an adequate width or a hemostatic dressing is sensible. Avoid overpacking with miles of half inch ribbon gauze; this is very painful to remove.

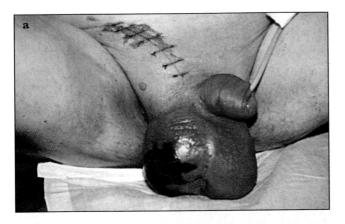

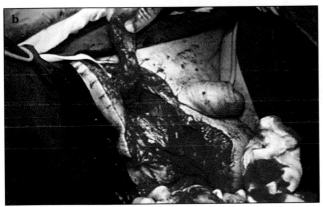

Figure 5.20 Necrotizing fasciitis before (a) and after (b) excision. Note that the skin changes are often the tip of the iceberg.

Necrotizing fasciitis

Although rare, it is important for the surgical resident to know about necrotizing fasciitis because a delay in the diagnosis and treatment will adversely influence survival. Categorization of necrotizing soft tissue infections is based on the anatomic level involved (skin, subcutaneous fat, fascia and skeletal muscle), the clinical picture and the infecting organisms. Clinical assessment alone is difficult. The anatomic level involved can only be determined at operation or microscopically, and multiple bacterial species may result in infections with an identical clinical appearance. These infections are important because they are capable of producing rapidly spreading soft tissue necrosis, severe systemic toxicity and high mortality. Early antibiotic therapy with broad-spectrum antibiotics such as penicillin, gentamycin and Flagyl is essential. Antibiotic therapy should be prescribed after discussion with the microbiology department.

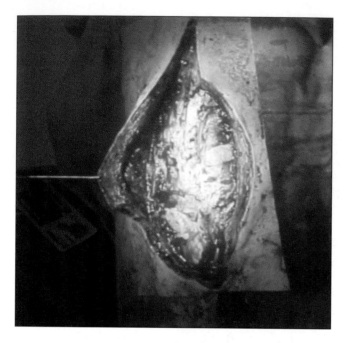

Figure 5.21 Abdominal wall debridement after clostridial infection.

Surgical exploration under general anesthetic is mandatory to determine the level of necrosis, to obtain pus and tissue for bacteriological analysis, to drain pus and to excise necrotic tissue. Multiple surgical procedures may be necessary to control the disease. Vigorous fluid resuscitation and cardiopulmonary support are just as important as the surgical therapy.

Gas gangrene caused by clostridial species is rarely seen outside trauma cases and is associated with the production of gas, causing crepitus.

Necrotizing fasciitis Type 1 (Fournier's gangrene) involves the scrotum, perineum, penis (see Figure 5.20) and abdominal wall (see Figure 5.21). The portal of entry is usually well defined and arises from anorectal/genitourinary infections and trauma (including surgery). The risk of developing necrotizing fasciitis is greater if the patient is diabetic, elderly and/or has co-existing cardiac and renal disease. In all patients with sepsis in this area, look for purple, gangrenous skin, particularly if other risk factors are present. Remember that the cutaneous component is 'the tip of the iceberg'. The testes, glans penis, bladder and rectum are usually spared because of their separate blood supplies. Causative organisms are mixed anaerobes and Gram-negative aerobic bacilli and enterococci. Fecal diversion is frequently required.

Despite optimal medical and surgical management, the mortality rate in many series exceeds 40%. It is important to warn the patient about widespread excision and the possible need for a stoma. Knowledge that the scrotal wall skin will heal and that testes can survive and be re-implanted in the thighs can be very reassuring.

Necrotizing fasciitis Type 2 infections are caused by Group A streptococcus. This disease is associated with penetrating injury, surgery, childbirth and blunt trauma. The disease causes marked swelling and pain, and the overlying skin becomes maroon or violaceous then rapidly gangrenous. There are marked systemic symptoms which include shock and organ failure.

chapter 6

Vascular emergencies

Mohammed Baguneid & Vince Smyth

Abdominal aortic aneurysm

An aneurysm can be defined as an 'abnormal localized dilatation of an artery'. As an abdominal aortic aneurysm (AAA) enlarges, the wall of the vessel weakens and there is an increasing risk of rupture. This risk is much greater if the aneurysm is 5.5 cm or greater on clinical examination; this is the threshold for elective repair. Pain and tenderness in the aneurysm are important warning signs of impending rupture. Following rupture, the leaking blood may be tamponaded by the region of the peritoneum anterior to the aorta, forming a hematoma. In this situation, a period of hemodynamic stability may occur. This is unpredictable in duration, typically a few hours at most, and will inevitably be followed by loss of tamponade and intraperitoneal blood loss if not treated urgently. If the blood is not contained by the peritoneum, loss is massive and few patients survive.

* the majority of patients (80%) with a ruptured AAA die without reaching hospital
* approximately 30–40% of those patients who make it to hospital die without reaching theater
* operative mortality is approximately 50%, this is usually due to multiple system organ failure
* overall mortality is 90%

These figures are in stark contrast to the 5–8% mortality from elective repair. The chances of repair and recovery are greatest in patients who do not display obvious clinical signs and when blood loss is minimal.

Very experienced vascular surgeons have stated that "leaking or ruptured AAAs are always detectable clinically" (although a firm, tender, non-pulsatile mass may be found in overweight, hypotensive patients).

> ! The key point to remember is to look and feel.

Disaster scenario one

A 74-year-old man who has collapsed after a long coach journey is admitted to the accident and emergency (A&E) department. He is resuscitated with a cup of tea and examined by the casualty officer. The patient feels light-headed when he sits or stands. The abdomen is not specifically palpated for an aneurysm. An electrocardiogram (ECG) is normal and a diagnosis of vaso-vagal attack is made. The patient stays in A&E for an hour, feels a little better and is sent home. He is readmitted *in extremis* with severe abdominal pain and profound hypotension 8 hours later. He is examined by a different casualty officer who diagnoses a ruptured AAA. Despite attempts to resuscitate he exanguinates before any attempt at surgical repair can be made.

Comment

A patient who has not previously had a vaso-vagal attack is highly unlikely to start at the age of 74 years. Always be highly suspicious when treating elderly patients with 'collapse'. A reasonable history is almost always available; vaso-vagal attacks are rare and significant pathology is common. Always remember to specifically palpate the abdominal aorta.

The typical patient is male, about 70 years old, hypertensive and a smoker. The classical presentation of ruptured AAA is of severe abdominal pain radiating through to the lower back, associated with collapse or confusion. The patient is pale, sweaty and hypotensive and will have a blood pressure (BP) of 80–100 mmHg with tachycardia, reflecting hypovolemia. Check for groin pulses, more distal pulses may be impalpable due to hypovolemia.

> ! Any patient over the age of 50 who collapses with back pain should be considered to have an AAA until proved otherwise.

Misdiagnosis of a leaking or ruptured AAA results in a very high risk of sudden death. When examining an emergency patient with a tender aneurysm it is safer for the surgical resident to assume that the aneurysm is the acute problem rather than seeking direct proof of leak or rupture on radiological grounds or by the development of profound hypotension.

> ! The role of the surgical resident is to detect the presence of the ruptured aneurysm, resuscitate the patient and mobilize forces.

Establish venous access with two large bore cannula and give fluid to maintain a systolic BP of 100 mmHg. Initiate cardiac and BP monitoring, give oxygen by facemask and insert a urethral catheter. Arrange an urgent full blood count and urea and electrolytes. A formal ECG and chest x-ray are not routinely required. Speak to the transfusion laboratory; initially request 8 units and warn them about the possible requirement for large quantities of blood and clotting products. If all parameters are normal, infuse crystalloid. If the patient is pale, sweaty and hypotensive, administer blood or colloid.

> ! Aim for a systolic BP of 80–100 mmHg; do not attempt to restore 'normal' BP as this may lead to loss of tamponade and rapid exsanguination.

You need to stay with the patient and monitor the effect of resuscitation. If blood is required it is better to wait until cross-matched blood is available. If the patient is improving with crystalloid continue with this but avoid large (2–3 L) transfusions with colloid as these will adversely affect clotting. O-negative blood, typed but uncross-matched, may be justified if hypotension is severe and the patient is not responding to colloid transfusion. The period and severity of hypotension are directly related to the chances of survival. Try to reserve some blood for theater.

A poor prognosis is associated with patients with pre-existing cardiac, respiratory or renal impairment prior to presentation, and patients requiring cardiopulmonary resuscitation in casualty.

Speak to the intensive care unit (ICU) staff and warn the theaters about the case. Even if the patient is stable ask for an urgent senior opinion. This is better than requesting an ultrasound examination because you are not in control of the amount of time taken for the test to be done and it is much harder to monitor the patient during transfer and performance of the scan. A portable ultrasound is occasionally valuable if there is diagnostic uncertainty. Ask for the old notes urgently. Some elderly patients with significant comorbidity will have been declared unfit for elective repair of an aneurysm.

Atypical presentations of a ruptured AAA include loin pain resembling renal colic, groin pain, hypotension, collapse with little in the way of abdominal pain, increased pain in an inguinal hernia and testicular pain. In all these situations, remember to look and feel for an aneurysm.

Disaster scenario two

A 74-year-old smoker is admitted at 11 am with a letter from his general practitioner requesting admission for investigation and management of his 'classical ureteric colic'. He has left-sided loin to groin pain which is not colicky in nature.

- pulse 90/minute
- BP 110/65 mmHg
- urinalysis, trace of blood
- tender left flank and left iliac fossa
- a kidney, ureter and bladder (KUB) scan shows linear calcification running in the line of the ureter overlying the transverse processes of L3 and L4
- past history of myocardial infarction (MI) with intermittent claudication, but no urolithiasis

The pre-registration house officer phones to say that the patient is comfortable after 100 mg of pethidine and that he is sending the patient to the ward. He has an intravenous urogram (IVU) that afternoon which the radiology specialist registrar provisionally reports as showing 'no left ureteric stone'. He requires further analgesia and feels unwell. He is reassessed but not examined and further pethidine is administered. At 11 pm he collapses.

- pulse 125/minute
- BP 80/50 mmHg
- abdomen distended and generally tender
- he is fully resuscitated and blood cross-matched
- at laparotomy an intraperitoneal AAA leak is found and dealt with

Comment

Any patient in the age group for cardiovascular diseases should be treated as having an aneurysm until positively proven otherwise. A trace of blood is not diagnostic of hematuria. It is rare for 74 year olds to have their first episode of ureteric colic.

His KUB shows calcification in the wall of the aneurysm (see Figure 6.01). If a patient has an unexpected result on an investigation one should ask why. His IVU request card had the words '? left ureteric colic' written on it. This report indicates that ureteric colic is not the cause of the illness. Better information could have helped steer the radiologist in the right direction, e.g. 'left loin pain, not classically colicky, linear calcification on KUB, smoker, previous MI'. The better the request information, the better the interpretation of the films will be.

If an investigation is important enough to carry out on the day of admission and the result does not fit in with the expected diagnosis, it is sensible to look at the films with a more senior clinician or radiologist as soon as possible.

When speaking to patients and relatives, tell them that a large blood vessel has ruptured in the abdomen and that without operation death is inevitable. You should alert relatives to the fact that the operation carries a mortality of up to 70% and that the patient will require postoperative high dependency unit or ICU care and will be critically ill for an undetermined period of time. Some families will decline surgery and some units may have protocols regarding suitability for operation, so to avoid distress tread carefully until the decision regarding surgery has been made. The final decision will usually be made by the consultant. Explain to the patient that they are likely to need to go to the ICU after the operation.

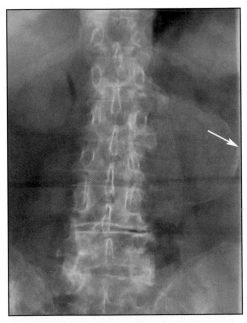

Figure 6.01 Calcification in the wall of an abdominal aortic aneurysm (arrow).

Acute limb ischemia

The two principal causes of acute ischemia are embolism and thrombosis (see Figure 6.02). The leg is affected by both, but upper limb ischemia almost always has an embolic etiology. When a vessel is occluded acutely the degree of ischemia is principally determined by collateral circulation. There is no time for a collateral circulation to develop with emboli so the ischemia will be severe. With thrombosis superimposed on existing peripheral vascular disease, there is a greater likelihood of a better developed collateral circulation, so ischemia may be less severe (see Figure 6.03).

Suspect an embolus if one of the following is present:

- atrial fibrillation
- good contralateral pulses
- recent MI, this may be silent so always perform an ECG
- valvular heart disease
- aortic aneurysm

Suspect a thrombus if one of the following is present:

- a history of claudication – the claudicant limb may not be the limb with the acute thrombus
- typical risk factors for arteriosclerosis – male, elderly, smokers, hypertensive patients
- previous bypass surgery for arteriosclerosis
- previous thrombosis
- young women on the contraceptive pill – occasionally these patients will present with *de novo* arterial thrombosis
- thrombophilia such as protein S deficiency or factor V Leiden mutation – these patients have poorly developed collaterals and ischemia may therefore be more acute

If a medical student is asked for the cardinal features of acute limb ischemia, a typical response is: **pallor, pulseless, painful, paralysis, paresthesia and perishing cold.**

If these features are placed in order of importance the list would be: **paralysis, paresthesia, pain, pulseless, perishing cold and pallor**.

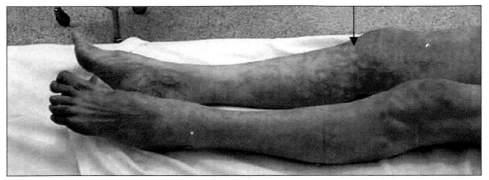

Figure 6.02 Acute lower limb ischemia (arrow).

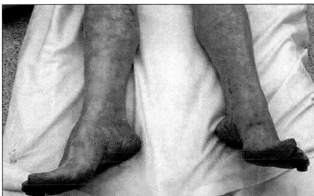

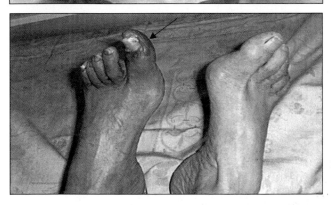

Figure 6.03 Critical limb ischemia on a background of lower limb vascular disease (arrow).

The value of thinking of the problem in this way is that in a limb of dubious viability, any degree of paralysis or paresthesia is highly significant and an indication that ischemia is severe. If rapid restoration of blood flow is not achieved, permanent neurological loss will occur. If the examining doctor spends time determining whether the leg is quite cold or perishing cold, or if a faint posterior tibial pulse can be felt, then the neurological examination may be neglected. It may only be a matter of hours before ischemia is irreversible. Note that acute swelling is almost never a feature of ischemia. In addition to the above, feel the consistency of the calf muscles and the degree of tenderness.

> **!** Fixed mottling, tender muscles and paralysis suggest irreversible ischemia.

Restoration of blood flow may cause systemic organ injury from reperfusion syndrome so primary amputation may be required. Take a full history of cardiac, cerebrovascular and peripheral vascular symptoms such as angina, MI, transient ischemic attack, stroke, claudication or cardiovascular surgery prior to this episode. Check for antiplatelet and anticoagulant medication and compliance. Ask about risk factors such as hypertension, diabetes or smoking.

Examine the cardiovascular system with particular reference to the appearance of the limb, palpable pulses and neurological status. Always examine both legs. A hand-held Doppler is invaluable for difficult to feel pulses. Document this with the time and date of examination.

Once a diagnosis of acute limb ischemia has been made, give 5000 international units (IU) of IV heparin. This buys some time for investigation and treatment. The speed of investigation and intervention depends on the degree of ischemia and the facilities available. Formal heparinization (1000 IU/hour IV) should be followed by a plan of action depending on the severity of presentation of the disease (see Table 6.01).

Grade	Clinical presentation	Action plan
I	No sensorimotor loss	Angiography on next elective list
IIa	Early sensory loss	Angiography ASAP, consider thrombolysis
IIb	Early motor loss	Surgical exploration with on-table angiography
III	Established motor loss	Analgesia, amputation on elective list

Table 6.01 Treatment of ischemia following heparinization depends on the severity of the disease.

If a confident diagnosis of embolus is made, it is safe to proceed directly to embolectomy. If the surgeon is experienced this can be performed under local anesthetic.

The diagnosis of acute graft failure postoperatively or deterioration in a patient having thrombolytic therapy is often difficult. Concerns are often raised late at night when the light on the ward is poor and the patient is not particularly cooperative. Read the operation note and the medical notes. Acute graft occlusion is more likely if the distal anastomosis is to a small vessel, there is poor run-off or if there have been technical difficulties during the procedure. It may even say in the notes: "Please inform me if there are concerns about graft patency."

Is the patient anticoagulated and has the patient been receiving anticoagulants? If there is uncertainty about anticoagulation, check the appropriate clotting parameters. Examine the affected limb and compare it with the normal limb. It is important to determine whether there is a pulse distal to the graft. If there is a clear Doppler signal at two points along the graft, the graft is patent. Always compare the Doppler signal with a readily palpable pulse to check you are hearing an arterial pulse rather than venous flow or an artifact. Check that the patient is generally well-oxygenated and perfused.

> **!** If you think a graft may have occluded then it probably has.

The long-term success of an acutely occluded graft depends on the speed with which it is unblocked, surgically or by lysis. Left untreated overnight, the ischemia may become irreversible. If you cannot be certain about graft patency or limb viability, ask for a senior opinion.

Compartment syndrome

Following reperfusion of an ischemic limb or organ there may be a reperfusion induced injury, i.e. exacerbation of the injury caused by the humoral and cellular components of acute inflammation. This results in damage to the endothelial lining of vessels in the ischemic tissue which become 'leaky' causing fluid accumulation in the extracellular space. Accumulation of osmotically active products of ischemic metabolism also increases fluid in the reperfused tissue.

In the calf, because of the enclosing fascial layers, the swelling may produce a rise in tissue pressure that exceeds the perfusion pressure of the newly restored circulation and this creates further ischemia. The blood flow in the major arteries is not affected until the compartment pressure rises to match systolic levels.

> **!** Thus further ischemia may occur even in the presence of palpable pulses.

If the high pressure in the compartment is not relieved by fasciotomy then permanent muscle damage and loss of the limb may occur. Note that compartment syndromes can occur after thrombolysis as well as embolectomy.

> **!** Compartment syndromes should be suspected in any reperfused limb with worsening pain, tenderness, swelling and sensory or motor loss.

It is sufficient for the surgical resident to be aware of the possibility of compartment syndrome and urgently alert a more senior colleague. Be aware that compartment syndromes can occur after prolonged operations in the lithotomy position. Remote organ injury may also occur as a result of the reperfusion syndrome with leaky capillaries in the lungs causing respiratory distress. Myoglobin release from muscle impairs renal function.

False aneurysm

A false aneurysm connects with the lumen of the artery but its outer wall is a hematoma confined by the adjacent tissues. The surgical resident sees false aneurysms most commonly at the puncture site after arteriography, at the site of vascular anastomosis and in drug addicts who inject into the femoral vessels. A small non-expanding false aneurysm, seen after arteriography, can safely be observed until review by the vascular team the following day. These can sometimes be treated by ultrasound-guided compression or by injection with bovine thrombin. Any false aneurysm observed in association with a vascular anastomosis and any expanding aneurysm should be discussed urgently with the vascular surgeons.

Most surgeons will know of cases where an unsuspecting surgical resident has confidently plunged a scalpel into the swollen red indurated groin of a drug addict expecting to release pus only to find a jet of blood passing his eyes and hitting the operating light. This produces a dangerous, uncontrolled and very embarrassing problem. Deep vein thrombosis and false aneurysms are common in IV drug addicts who inject into the groin so for these patients always arrange an ultrasound scan. The scan will show the presence and position of pus, which may be deep in the vessel and, therefore, may not easily be drained surgically. Ultrasound-guided drainage may be possible. If the scan does confirm pus anterior to the vessels and normal femoral vessels then the knife can be confidently applied.

chapter 7

Trauma

Ajith Siriwardena & James Hill

Managing the trauma patient is one of the most challenging and stressful problems for the surgical resident. Patients are often admitted late at night, they can be difficult to assess and may even be threatening at times. Stress levels are increased by the presence of police, paramedics and anxious relatives. Concentrate on basic resuscitation, followed by assessment of injuries and then definitive management. Since assessment of a patient may be difficult and deterioration rapid, do not hesitate in asking for a senior opinion. Attending an advanced trauma life support course is strongly recommended; this is mandatory for surgical residents in the UK.

Penetrating injury – stab wounds

Neck

Any penetrating wound where there is compromise of an airway, an expanding hematoma, uncontrollable hemorrhage or shock should be explored.

Chest

The majority (75–85%) of penetrating chest wounds can be effectively treated using a chest drain. A thoracotomy will be required by 10–15% after a secondary examination. A small number, around 5%, will require an immediate thoracotomy. An example of a chest stab wound is provided in Figure 7.01.

Management of a chest stab wound differs depending on the condition of the patient. Stable patients should have a chest x-ray (CXR). If this shows a hemothorax or a pneumothorax, insert a chest drain and arrange a repeat CXR. If the pneumothorax has resolved or the bleeding has stopped after the second CXR, then simple observation is sufficient.

Unstable patients should be given oxygen. Arrange a portable CXR, insert an intravenous (IV) line, send blood to be cross-matched, insert a Foley catheter and consult senior help. Investigations for patients not requiring an immediate thoracotomy include arteriography and computed tomography (CT) scanning. Parasternal wounds are associated with an increased risk of cardiac injuries. Cardiac tamponade can be

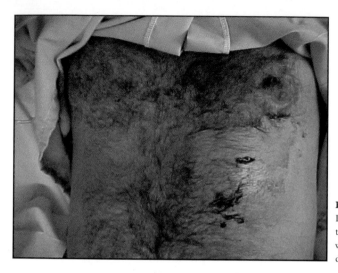

Figure 7.01 Stab wound to the chest. Injury to thoracic, abdominal organs and the diaphragm are likely. Penetrating wounds around this site pose great danger.

rapidly fatal. The signs (Beck's triad) of hypotension, muffled heart sound and a raided jugular venous pressure are difficult to assess and not always present. Seek immediate senior assistance for any patient with a penetrating parasternal wound.

Abdominal

Patients fall into one of three categories:

- wound with associated peritonitis or hypotension – laparotomy required
- superficial wound – local treatment required
- wound of uncertain depth without peritonitis or hypotension – management depends on clinical/radiological findings and local protocols

There is an increasing trend towards conservative management of penetrating injuries. In parts of the world where an immense amount of penetrating trauma is seen, such as in South Africa, this pragmatic approach is necessary to cope with the volume of cases. In the UK, where penetrating trauma is relatively uncommon, there is a greater tendency to explore wounds under a general anesthetic, with examination of the peritoneal cavity if the peritoneum has been breached. Some surgeons advocate mandatory operation for any potentially penetrating wound and accept that this will lead to negative laparotomies.

If a conservative approach is adopted, a repeat clinical examination is necessary to look for any increase in abdominal tenderness and distension, and changes in the pulse and blood pressure (BP). A CT or ultrasound scan, serial measurement of hemoglobin and a white blood cell (WBC) count may provide reassurance for a continued conservative approach.

- penetrating injuries do not respect anatomical boundaries. Stab wounds between the nipples and umbilicus commonly produce thoraco-abdominal injuries
- one-third of anterior abdominal stab wounds do not penetrate the peritoneal cavity
- of those that penetrate the peritoneal cavity less than half cause significant visceral injury
- the risk of visceral injury is approximately 10% for penetrating wounds to the back and approximately 25% for penetrating wounds to the flank

It is safe to explore stab wounds in the accident and emergency (A&E) department to determine the depth. After infiltration with local anesthetic, retract the wound edges and examine in good light. If the deep extent of the wound can be seen, and the peritoneum is not breached, conservative treatment is appropriate.

With penetrating stab wounds look for the following warning signs:

- parasternal wounds
- wounds between the nipple and umbilicus
- hypotension
- dyspnea
- peritonitis

Disaster scenario

A 26-year-old man is admitted at 2 am with a stab wound to the epigastrium which occurred 1 hour earlier. The mechanism of injury and the weapon used could not be determined. No other injuries were sustained.

Examination
- pulse 90/minute
- BP 120/80 mmHg
- there is a 2 cm entry wound in the epigastrium, it is not possible to determine the depth of the wound, no visible external blood loss

- abdominal tenderness with guarding from the xiphisternum to the level of the umbilicus
- hemoglobin (Hb) 10.9 g/dL
- blood is cross-matched and 4 units are requested

The case is discussed with the higher surgical trainee (HST) who agrees to examine the patient. The HST falls asleep and is woken by the basic surgical trainee at 3 am. The pulse and BP have been stable during this hour. The HST advises that, as the patient is stable, conservative therapy should be continued with observation. No investigations are advised. The patient remains in A&E due to a shortage of ward beds. The following day a new surgical team come on duty; no advice is given about the patient. At 11 am the on-call surgical resident is urgently alerted as the patient has become hypotensive (BP 80/50 mmHg) and tachycardic (pulse 120/minute). He is now found to have generalized abdominal tenderness.

On emergency laparotomy, 2 L of intraperitoneal free blood, laceration of left lobe of the liver and penetrating parenchymal injury to the pancreas are discovered.

Comment

Every attempt must be made to find as much information as possible about the weapon used and the mechanism of injury. In the absence of this information, it must be assumed that the knife was very long and very sharp! The mechanism of injury is equally important and will give important clues about the likely depth of penetration and which organs are likely to have been injured.

The initial management of this case has been reasonable given that the patient was stable, the Hb level and the fact that the tenderness was localized. However, there is a suspicion that the peritoneal cavity has been breached and the reduced Hb level in this patient only 1 hour after the stab wound suggests significant blood loss. The surgical resident should insist that the HST sees the patient. If an attempt at conservative treatment is made then initially a 1–2 hourly review would be required rather than the 8 hours that elapsed. The surgical resident must ensure that adequate hand-over arrangements are made when no longer on duty and he or she should speak directly to the next duty team about worrying cases.

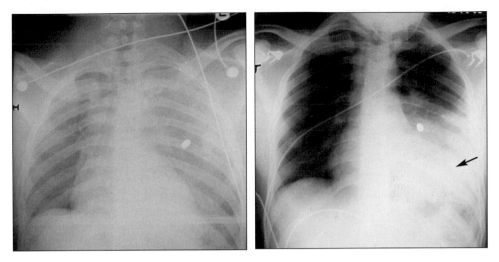

Figure 7.02 Chest x-ray of a patient with a bullet wound to the left hemothorax: (a) in the supine view the hemothorax cannot be seen; (b) an erect x-ray is required whenever a hemothorax is suspected (arrow).

Penetrating injury – bullet wounds

In the UK, bullet wounds are rare. The risks of significant visceral injury are higher than those for stab wounds. The surgical resident should ask for immediate senior help to manage these patients. An example of a chest bullet wound is provided in figure 7.02.

Blunt trauma

Severe abdominal blunt trauma is uncommon in the UK. Abdominal injury is frequently associated with other injuries. Examples of abdominal seat belt trauma and secondary injury to the small bowel are provided in Figures 7.03 and 7.04. Altered levels of consciousness from head injury, severe pain from soft tissue and orthopedic injuries make clinical assessment of the abdomen difficult. Indeed patients are frequently intubated and ventilated before being seen by the surgical team. The other systemic parameters used to assess intra-abdominal pathology, such as pulse and temperature, are also affected by other injuries. For the severely injured patient the surgical resident should not make an assessment alone. Any decision should involve a more senior surgeon.

Clear indications for laparotomy include free intraperitoneal gas, hemodynamic shock not explained by other injuries, rupture of the diaphragm and intraperitoneal

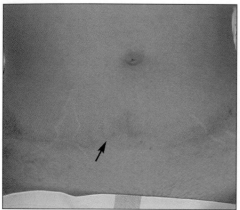

Figure 7.03 Seat belt trauma to the abdominal wall (arrow).

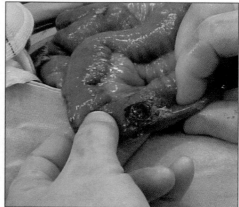

Figure 7.04 Secondary small bowel perforation as a result of seat belt trauma.

rupture of the bladder. In the absence of laparoscopy (this technique may not be available in many centers) or if no clear indications for laparotomy are present on first assessment, appropriate investigations include CT scanning, ultrasound scanning and peritoneal lavage. Laparoscopy should only be performed by an experienced surgeon.

CT scan

This is highly accurate and will detect as little as 10 cc of free fluid and parenchymal injury to all solid organs in the abdomen. It is much less effective at diagnosing rupture of the gastrointestinal tract. Another major advantage of CT scanning is that several sites can be examined in a short period of time. With spiral CT scanning it is possible to scan the head, cervical spine, chest, abdomen and pelvis in a few minutes.

Ultrasound scan

In good hands, ultrasound scanning of the abdomen is comparable to CT scanning. Detection of injury to luminal organs is less accurate and examination of retroperitoneal structures is not as easy as with CT scanning.

Diagnostic peritoneal lavage

A peritoneal dialysis catheter is placed into the peritoneal cavity in the subumbilical position under local anesthetic. It is usually performed in A&E after the period of initial resuscitation. If fresh blood or enteric contents can be aspirated directly or the lavage return is grossly bloody, then laparotomy is indicated. If not, 1 L of normal saline is instilled into the peritoneal cavity. The fluid is then allowed to siphon back out passively into the infusion bag. This fluid should then be examined microscopically. If the red cell count is greater than 100,000 cells/mm^3 or the WBC count is greater than 500 cells/mm^3, laparotomy is performed. As a rough guide, if newspaper sized print cannot be read through the returned fluid then the red cell count will be above 100,000 cells/mm^3. The majority of patients with bowel injuries have an elevated WBC count in the lavage fluid. The test is also positive if the lavage fluid is seen passing into the chest drain or urethral catheter; surgical intervention is likely to be required. Peritoneal lavage is very accurate and may have an advantage over CT scanning for detecting bowel injuries. It also has a role in the absence of CT scanning facilities and where movement of the patient is contraindicated or presents logistic difficulties. Peritoneal lavage is probably the best test for diaphragmatic injury seen most commonly with penetrating thoraco-abdominal trauma. This form of injury shows no distinctive symptoms and signs. It is difficult to diagnose with laparoscopy and if not detected it is likely that it will present at a later date with obstruction or strangulation of abdominal viscera.

Splenic trauma

Suspect splenic injury when there has been a blow to the left side of the abdomen, especially when there are fractures of overlying ribs (ribs numbered 9, 10 or 11). Clinical signs are determined by the severity of the musculoskeletal injury and the amount of intraperitoneal blood loss. Whenever splenic trauma is suspected, check a full blood count and cross-match blood. If the patient has hypovolemic shock despite resuscitation then a laparotomy is required. If the patient is stable, an ultrasound or CT scan should be performed. Where possible, splenic conservation should be attempted. The injury may be treated conservatively without surgery if there is no major parenchymal injury or large quantity of free intraperitoneal blood.

The key to management is careful and frequent re-evaluation. Increasing pain and tenderness, persistent tachycardia and hypotension despite transfusion, ongoing transfusion requirements and a falling Hb level are all indications for surgical intervention. Attempts at splenic conservation can be made at laparotomy and are dependent on the severity of the injury. The risks of late bleeding after conservative nonoperative treatment are small. The value of retaining the spleen is to avoid the small risk of overwhelming post-splenectomy sepsis. If splenectomy has been performed then immunization against pneumococcus, hemophilus and meningococcus are necessary, as is treatment with oral penicillin.

Liver and biliary trauma

Blunt trauma to the liver is nearly always seen in patients with multiple injuries. CT scanning is the investigation of choice. Whenever a liver injury is detected ask for a senior opinion.

Renal trauma

Renal trauma scenario

A married couple are involved in a road traffic accident. While traveling at 35 mph they collide with a car coming out of a side road traveling at a similar speed. Both are wearing seat belts. They are examined in the trauma resuscitation room.

The husband has a bruise from his seat belt and is tender over the right upper quadrant. He is feeling unwell with a tachycardia of 120/minute and a BP of 105/60 mmHg. A diagnostic peritoneal lavage is negative. There is a small amount of blood detectable in his catheter specimen of urine.

His wife has a left-sided hematoma from where the door of the car hit her. She has pain over the bruise and in the left loin and has fractured her lower-most two ribs on the left side. Her pulse is 100/minute and her BP is 140/85 mmHg. She has frank hematuria and a negative diagnostic peritoneal lavage.

Negative peritoneal lavage results indicate that neither is likely to have an intraperitoneal injury. The location of the pain and bruising, combined with rib fractures and hematuria, indicate that both patients have renal injuries.

- who has the more severely injured kidney?
- who should be resuscitated first?
- what imaging technique should be used?
- who should be wheeled round to the radiology department first?
- how will their management differ?

On clinical assessment alone it is not possible to determine who has the more severe renal injury. The husband has a clinical picture fitting with an injury to the renal pedicle. This is an acceleration/deceleration injury. He is shocked and clearly needs aggressive resuscitation. A CT scan with contrast should be the imaging method of choice. This will confirm a right kidney with an affected blood supply displayed by poor uptake of contrast. This is the reason for the unimpressive amount of blood in his urine. Contrast CT will also show that the kidney on the other side is working. Surgical exploration is mandatory here. The kidney may be saved but it may require removal if bleeding cannot be controlled.

His wife is stable. She is likely to have a moderate degree of injury to her kidney with bleeding into the collecting system. In the absence of shock or an expanding hematoma, it is usual to be able to manage this injury conservatively. The ideal imaging technique again is a CT scan with contrast, however, a plain abdominal x-ray followed by IV contrast injection and a further film 10–20 minutes later may give enough information to allow you to safely manage this patient while attending to her husband.

The message is that the degree of hematuria does not necessarily correlate with the degree of the renal injury.

Vascular trauma

Vascular injury can be due to:

- penetrating trauma causing direct vascular damage
- blunt trauma resulting in vascular compression or creation of an intimal dissection flap

Whatever the cause, management essentially follows the guidelines described for acute limb ischemia. One exception is that if vascular compromise is associated with a displaced or fractured bone, then arterial investigation and management will often coincide with or follow urgent reduction and fixation of the orthopedic injury. In most cases an on-table angiogram is necessary.

chapter 8

Urological emergencies
Richard Napier-Hemy

Acute testicular pain

When a patient presents with acute testicular pain one of the following is likely:

- torsion of the testis
- acute epididymo-orchitis
- testicular tumor
- trauma
- torsion of the appendix testis
- idiopathic scrotal edema

Testicular torsion
Testicular torsion is the most important diagnosis to exclude. Every case of scrotal pain will be referred to you with a letter that says: "I cannot exclude testicular torsion." This condition is not the most common cause of scrotal pain but clearly it has the most severe consequences if missed.

> ! A scrotal exploration should always be performed unless a positive diagnosis excluding torsion can be made.

Acute epididymo-orchitis
Acute epididymo-orchitis is suggested by epididymal distension and tenderness greater than testicular swelling and tenderness. This may be associated with pyrexia, systemic signs and symptoms of sepsis, a urinalysis suggestive of infection, and an ultrasound scan (USS) Doppler that shows increased blood flow. Be aware that the twisted cord of the testicle can feel like a distended epididymis to the unwary.

Trauma
Trauma is usually suggested by the history. Expect there to be bruising and swelling so that the normal anatomy is not discernible. In the presence of an expanding hematoma, surgical exploration will be required. However, beware, because trauma can cause a testicle to tort or the history of trauma can be a red herring.

Testicular tumors

Testicular tumors usually present as a painless mass. Approximately 10% will present as an inflammatory mass with pain. They can be difficult to differentiate from infection. An USS with α-fetoprotein and β-human chorionic gonadotropin estimation will usually, though not always, clarify things. If a testicular tumor is suspected then any surgical exploration should be undertaken through a groin incision.

Torsion of the appendix testis

Torsion of the appendix testis or hydatid of Morgagni is the most common cause of acute testicular pain in a child. A clinical diagnosis can be made if the pain and tenderness are isolated to the upper pole of the testicle and the classical 'blue spot' sign can be seen through the scrotal skin. The blue spot can be difficult to see with darker scrotal skin. If this diagnosis can confidently be made, the patient can be managed conservatively and should be told that the pain should settle in a few days. If there is severe pain, or the pain fails to settle, then surgical excision of the torted appendix testis is the cure. However, the patient will have the pain and possible complications of an operation instead.

Idiopathic scrotal edema

Idiopathic scrotal edema is a rarity but will usually be referred to a surgical resident if identified. It is common in younger boys and can present with pain. The patient will have the appearance of bruising and edema over the scrotal skin and shaft of the penis. The testes should be palpable and should not be tender. Conservative management is the order of the day.

In the absence of another positive diagnosis, the patient should be treated as suffering from torsion of the testicle. A surgical exploration should be planned as soon as is safely possible. Your colleagues in other surgical specialties will understand that this potentially organ-saving procedure should not be delayed. Ideally, surgery should take place within 4–6 hours of the onset of pain. However, just because the pain has gone on longer does not mean that the testicle is dead and exploration can be delayed.

The patient and/or his parents should be informed that the operation is the best investigation available. An USS can be unreliable, particularly in children. Nuclear medicine perfusion scanning is not a viable proposition. The patient should be prepared for exploration and either fixation of the testicle or removal if the testicle is beyond redemption.

Renal/ureteric colic

The diagnosis of renal or ureteric calculus can usually be made confidently by the time the patient leaves the accident and emergency (A&E) department.

Expect patients to present with two, if not all, of the following three features:

- a classical history of colicky loin to groin pain
- hematuria, either macroscopic or more usually dipstick/microscopic
- a positive kidney, ureter and bladder (KUB) plain abdominal x-ray

If only one of the above is present then question the diagnosis of ureteric colic. There may be other features as well. The severe pain causes nausea and vomiting. Bowel dilatation can be seen on the x-ray. The patient may have lower urinary tract symptoms compatible with a lower urinary tract infection (UTI). This is more common if there is a stone within the intramural part of the ureter or at the ureterovesical junction. As the stone passes down or lodges in the ureter, pain can be experienced in the groin, suprapubic region and tip of the penis. A typical examination finding is tenderness in the line of the renal tract. Guarding and rebound tenderness are sometimes seen. These can be quite impressive but should settle if the patient's pain is appropriately managed. The presence of a renal mass suggests pyonephrosis, pelvi-ureteric junction (PUJ) obstruction, a cyst or tumor. A KUB x-ray shows a stone in 90% of cases. Examples of renal calculi are provided in Figures 8.01–8.04.

Investigation

- full blood count (FBC)
- urea and electrolytes (U&E)
- mid-stream urine (MSU)
- intravenous urography (IVU)

Management

- analgesia with pethidine as the opiate of choice. Nonsteroidal anti-inflammatory drugs such as diclofenac work well for ureteric colic and a good response to such analgesics supports the diagnosis of ureteric colic
- hydration with IV crystalloid is only required if the patient cannot tolerate oral fluids. Avoid the temptation of trying to flush the stone out with a vigorous diuresis. It is peristalsis that propels a stone down the ureter and not a head of fluid

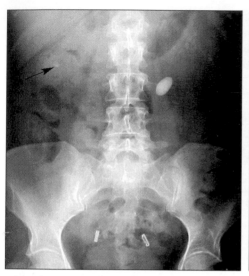

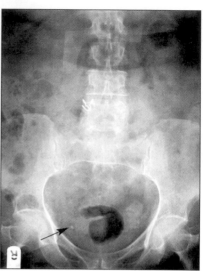

Figure 8.01 A kidney, ureter and bladder x-ray showing a large left renal pelvic calculus sitting in the pelvi-ureteric junction. Not all stones causing colic are this easy to spot. There are also calyceal calculi in the right kidney (arrow).

Figure 8.02 Right lower ureteric calculi can sometimes be mistaken for phleboliths. These are usually very round and often below the level of the ischial spines. This stone has some characteristics of a phlebolith but its long axis runs in the line of the ureter (arrow).

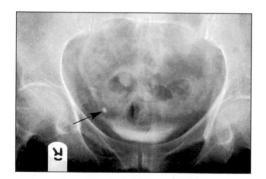

Figure 8.03 Sometimes the only way of telling whether an opacity is a stone or a phlebolith is with intravenous urography. This confirms the opacity to be in the line of the ureter (arrow). This is the same patient as in Figure 8.02.

If there is a clinical suspicion of infection proximal to the stone (particularly if the patient has a single functioning kidney), an urgent ultrasound scan is mandatory. An obstructed infected kidney needs drainage with a nephrostomy after administration of parenteral antibiotics. This should be done urgently as untreated pyonephrosis has

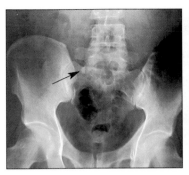 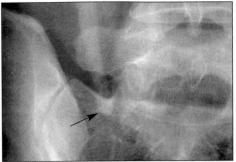

Figure 8.04 If the story and urinalysis strongly point to the likelihood of ureteric colic then the stone may either be radiolucent or over a bony prominence (arrows). The intravenous urogram reveals an opacity just medial to the upper end of the sacro-iliac joint causing partial obstruction.

a high mortality rate, particularly in already frail patients. An acutely obstructed kidney may not have had time to develop a significant hydronephrosis. Thus, clinical fears must be made clear to the radiologist. If an ultrasound scan fails to give information regarding the clinical suspicion of infection and obstruction, then an IVU or a renogram is appropriate to establish that the kidney is functioning and draining. An IVU is more likely to be available in an emergency.

Disaster scenario one

A 25-year-old woman is referred by her general practitioner (GP) with a 2-week history of right loin pain, a history of rigors and had been taking oral antibiotics. Today she has started vomiting and feels much more unwell. She arrives in A&E at 8 pm.

On examination she has a temperature of 39.8°C, a pulse of 125/minute and a blood pressure (BP) of 100/60 mmHg. She is dehydrated and has a very tender right loin. An MSU result shows pyuria but no bacteria.

Action taken
- blood cultures
- analgesia
- oral antibiotics
- a KUB x-ray that shows no stone

On the post-take ward round the patient is sleeping and is not disturbed. The nursing staff try to rouse her 2 hours later. She is drowsy, confused, cyanosed and has a purpuric rash. The medical staff are urgently alerted.

Action taken
- full resuscitation with an ABC approach
- oxygen
- IV access and IV fluids
- parenteral antibiotics
- arterial blood gases show hypoxia and severe metabolic acidosis
- elevated creatinine
- intensive treatment unit (ITU) admission required with respiratory and renal support
- ultrasound scan shows thin cortex and gross hydronephrosis
- percutaneous nephrostomy drains 300 mL of pus

Comment

The patient's background history raises the possibility of a PUJ obstruction. This young lady was very unwell at the time of admission and required more aggressive treatment at that time. Her MSU shows a 'sterile pyuria' and is likely to show this because the MSU was sent when she was already on antibiotics. However, complete obstruction can prevent white blood cells and bacteria from reaching the bladder and being found in the MSU. Because of her history, and the degree of systemic upset, an early ultrasound scan with a view to nephrostomy insertion would be reasonable. Even with early nephrostomy insertion there is still a chance that she would have required either ITU or high dependency unit admission.

Acute pyelonephritis

As with renal colic, the diagnosis of upper renal tract infection is usually readily made. The combination of dysuria, frequency, loin pain, pyrexia and rigors is seen in most patients; nausea and vomiting are common. Typical patients are young women, patients with pre-existing renal disease and those with a previous history of urinary infection. On examination the patient is flushed and tachycardic with a high fever and marked tenderness over the infected kidney. The main differential diagnoses are renal colic, acute appendicitis and acute biliary problems.

Investigation

- FBC
- U&E
- MSU must be sent
- dipstick urinalysis showing leukocytes, nitrates, protein and blood strongly supports the diagnosis of acute pyelonephritis and can probably replace urgent microscopy
- blood cultures
- an USS during admission to exclude obstruction – this is preferred to IVU as infection and the contrast medium are both slightly nephrotoxic

Following treatment with appropriate antibiotics, the pain and temperature should start to settle within 24 hours, but it may take several days before the patient becomes apyrexial. Chase the MSU result, this may be available within 24 hours. If positive, it will confirm the diagnosis and help in choosing an appropriate antibiotic. If the clinical condition and temperature do not improve then expedite the ultrasound appointment to exclude an abscess or pyonephrosis and consider a change of antibiotics. Fecal streptococci can cause a UTI and will often be sensitive to amoxicillin.

Management

- IV rehydration
- IV antibiotics – the most common organisms encountered are coliforms, proteus and pseudomonads. Suitable antibiotics are aminoglycosides such as gentamicin, 5 mg/kg as a single daily infusion, or quinolones, such as norfloxacin or ciprofloxacin. The choice of antibiotic will probably depend on local prescribing protocols and whether or not parenteral antibiotics are required

Acute retention of urine

Acute retention of urine is one of the most common surgical emergencies. Diagnosis should not present any great difficulty. The bladder should be easily palpable with the upper border close to the umbilicus. The patient should be in pain or at least discomfort. It is kind to catheterize the patient promptly to relieve discomfort before taking a full history. Digital rectal examination should certainly be performed with an empty bladder as otherwise the size of the prostate can be overestimated. For a man, a size 14 F or 16 F soft, short-term catheter should be inserted using aseptic technique.

Female patients should ideally have a 12 F catheter. Remember to record the volume of urine drained as this information is of prognostic value and will be used by the urological team to plan future management. A residual of over 800 mL implies that there has been a longstanding lower urinary tract problem. These patients have a lower chance of voiding on removal of their catheter. Failure to insert the catheter is usually due to either urethral stricture or obstruction at the level of the prostate gland. Patients with a urethral stricture may have a previous history. If the urethral catheter can only be passed a few cm then a urethral stricture is likely. Insertion of a catheter with a smaller diameter can be gently attempted. If the obstruction is at the level of the prostate gland then a size 16 coude can be tried. The curvature at the tip of this catheter aids passage through the prostatic urethra. After two failed attempts a surgical resident should seek help from someone more experienced. If catheterization has not been easy then a single dose of antibiotics such as a quinolone or gentamicin is sensible. If urethral catheterization is not possible, the bladder is palpable and there is no history to raise the suspicion of a bladder tumor being present, then a suprapubic catheter should be inserted. If you have not inserted a suprapubic catheter before then ensure that you perform this with an experienced assistant.

! The surgical resident should never be tempted to use a catheter introducer.

Beware of the patient who is sent with a diagnosis of acute retention of urine but who, when catheterized, produces only a small volume of concentrated urine. This is a common mode of presentation for patients with lower abdominal peritonitis. Always check that catheterization has cured the suprapubic pain, tenderness and mass to avoid being caught out.

Most patients nowadays opt for a trial without catheter. Those with large residual volumes and/or large prostate glands are less likely to pass this trial.

Catheterization and acute urinary retention can cause plasma prostate specific antigen (PSA) levels to elevate. There is no place for routine PSA estimation at the time of emergency admission.

Acute retention of urine is rare in women and should be dealt with in the same way as for men. Urethral catheterization rarely fails. Exclude pregnancy before contemplating a suprapubic catheterization. Investigation at a later date will be aimed at establishing whether there is an intravesical, mural or pelvic space-occupying lesion present, or whether there are drug effects or a neurological condition.

Disaster scenario two

An 81-year-old man is sent to hospital from a nursing home with a history of:

- 18-hour anuria
- suprapubic pain
- suprapubic mass
- recent diarrhea
- confusion
- fever

The letter from his GP said: "could you sort out this usually sprightly octogenarian who has developed urinary retention secondary to a UTI?"

He is assessed at 4 am, a full history is taken and an examination is performed. He is catheterized with ease and clear urine drains. The pre-registration house officer is called to A&E and writes the notes hurriedly. The house officer informs the surgical resident when they meet each other in A&E.

At 6.30 am the nursing staff call the surgical resident to say that the patient has a BP of 95/45 mmHg and is more confused. A saline drip is started. The house officer reassesses him and queries whether the bladder is still palpable. The catheter has only drained 200 mL. The catheter is flushed and some urine starts to drain. His BP is now 110/55 mmHg.

On the post-take ward round at 8.30 am he is re-examined by the specialist registrar. The patient is drowsy following opiate analgesia. His total urine output since catheterization has been 250 mL. The bladder is no longer palpable but his abdomen seems to be slightly tender all over.

At 9 am he is seen by the consultant surgeon. His BP is 85/50 mmHg. He is unwell and tachycardic, with signs of generalized peritonitis. He is resuscitated with fluids, given broad-spectrum antibiotics and a laparotomy is arranged. At operation he is found to have a pelvic abscess, probably originally caused by a localized large bowel pathology. This has burst into the peritoneal cavity.

Comment

Symptoms of anuria, suprapubic pain and a suprapubic mass do not always mean acute urinary retention. If the residual had been recorded, and the patient re-examined after catheterization, then the surgical resident would have realized that there must be some other pathology. This would have altered the patient's management which should have been more aggressive, focusing on diagnosis and treatment of the cause of the intra-abdominal mass. The surgical resident should have asked the house officer the following two questions:

- what was the residual?
- did the catheter sort out the pain, tenderness and mass?

If the residual was unknown then one of the ward staff could have been contacted from A&E.

Chronic urinary retention

If the patient has no pain or tenderness but has a palpable bladder then do not rush to insert a catheter. Such patients are likely to have either low pressure or high pressure chronic retention. Low pressure chronic retention is caused by failure of the detrusor muscle to contract adequately to empty the bladder. The pressure in the bladder is low and the presence of a large residual urine does not necessarily require treatment. However, the residual urine can have undesirable consequences.

Any of the following should be investigated:

- UTI
- intolerable urinary frequency
- stone disease
- incontinence
- obstructive uropathy

High pressure chronic retention is caused by outlet obstruction. Hydronephrosis and evidence of renal failure will be present. The patient will eventually need some permanent form of management such as transurethral resection of the prostate.

Management of painless retention

- check creatinine and electrolytes
- catheterize if potassium is elevated
- if creatinine is above 300 mmol/L consider catheterization. This should probably be discussed with a urologist and can often wait until the next morning
- after catheterization expect a post-obstructive diuresis and hematuria. The patient will need close monitoring to ensure that there is not too much fluid loss

Monitor
- daily creatinine and electrolytes
- daily weight
- erect and supine BP
- fluid input and output chart
- if signs of excessive diuresis are evident then give normal saline by IV infusion
- urological referral and an ultrasound scan of the kidneys will be required

Penile problems

Phimosis
A tight prepuce can prevent adequate cleansing of the glans penis and can lead to infection. This is most often seen in children and can cause such pain that the patient is reluctant to void.

Phimosis can cause acute urinary retention. The hole through the prepuce will be tiny. Circumcision, dorsal slit of the prepuce or suprapubic catheter insertion will relieve the obstruction. All of these can, with appropriate experience, be performed under local anesthesia.

Paraphimosis
This condition develops when a tight foreskin is retracted over the glans penis for a prolonged period of time. It cannot be brought forward and causes swelling of the glans. When first called about this problem advise the referring team to apply ice-filled gloves to the penis to try to decrease the swelling. Reduction requires the coordination of two maneuvers. Firstly the glans should be gently squeezed for a few minutes under appropriate analgesia. When the swelling has decreased, the prepuce is advanced at the same time that the glans is pushed through the constriction

ring of the prepuce. If manual reduction fails then emergency circumcision or dorsal slit will be required.

Priapism

Prolonged erection is usually caused by the injection of vasoactive drugs used in the management of erectile dysfunction. This urological emergency will require the involvement of more experienced staff. Spontaneous priapism may be caused by a hematological condition such as sickle disease or leukemia. If a patient presents with a spontaneous priapism then make sure that a FBC and U&E are performed. If there is an underlying cause then it must be addressed. The priapism may require treatment with aspiration of blood though a large bore cannula and intracorporal administration of vasoconstrictors such as phenylephrine or metaraminol. Surgery may be required so the patient should be kept starved. High-flow priapism, where the blood flow into the penis is increased, may require angiography and embolization.

Catheter problems

Indwelling urinary catheters, suprapubic or urethral, cause a variety of problems that can present at A&E (see Table 8.01).

Problem	Action
Blockage	Change the catheter – once a catheter is coated and blocked, flushing it will not work for very long
Bypassing	Check that the catheter is not blocked – if it is draining well then bypassing can be caused by detrusor contractions. Exclude a UTI. Remove some water from the catheter balloon. Administer antimuscarinics such as oxybutynin or tolterodine. Change the catheter for a smaller, less irritating one
Expulsion	Treat as for bypassing but question whether there should be a change in the management plan. A suprapubic catheter may suit the patient better but should not be put in by the inexperienced in this situation. It may even require general anesthetic or open insertion
Hematuria	Exclude infection. Never assume that the hematuria is caused by the catheter. Full investigation is reasonable
Recurrent UTI	Send catheter urine specimens for microscopy. Culture and sensitivity tests. Increase fluids. Change the catheter? Antibiotic prophylaxis. Consider an investigation to look for stones or upper tract pathologies

Table 8.01 Common problems with catheters.

Hematuria

Frank hematuria is a worrying symptom and demands a full investigation, particularly in patients over the age of 40 years when the incidence of urothelial cancer increases. Hematuria rarely requires emergency admission, although many patients will either be referred by their GP or self-present. Most patients can be managed at home with urgent investigations arranged on an out-patient basis.

Investigation

- MSU
- cytology
- FBC
- U&E
- urgent IVU
- cystoscopy

Criteria for emergency admission

- shock
- anemia
- clot retention
- pain
- inability to cope at home

Emergency management

- admit if one of the criteria for emergency admission is fulfilled
- check FBC
- examine to exclude clot retention
- send MSU
- advise the patient to increase fluid intake
- arrange an IVU

If there is no reason to admit then fax or hand deliver the A&E records to the urology office so that an appropriate urgent follow-up can be arranged.

Clot retention

This should be dealt with by insertion of a large (20–22 F) three-way silicone or simplastic urethral catheter. The bladder can be washed out through this to remove all clots. An USS can be useful for determining whether a clot remains present within the bladder. When the bladder is free of clots then irrigation with saline will help to stop the blood from clotting again.

chapter 9

Postoperative complications

Richard Bowman & James Hill

Some postoperative complications are inevitable. There is evidence that morbidity and mortality rates are reduced by managing high-risk patients in the high dependency unit (HDU).

The HDU provides:

- central venous pressure monitoring
- arterial line pressure recording and blood gas measurement
- pulse oximetry
- high-flow oxygen
- epidural management
- continuous positive airways pressure (CPAP)
- fluid balance and vital sign measurement
- electrocardiogram (ECG) monitoring
- skilled and experienced nursing staff who identify problems early

The HDU does not provide:

- intermittent positive pressure ventilation
- hemodialysis
- left atrial end diastolic pressure monitoring via a Swan-Ganz catheter

The HDU is ideal for high-risk surgical patients who are breathing spontaneously. The intensive care unit (ICU) is ideal for patients requiring ventilation, renal support or inotropic support. Any patient in the HDU needing CPAP or inotropes should be discussed with the ICU with a view to a possible transfer.

HDU care should be provided at the surgical resident level and above. Most units have good working relationships with anesthetists who are almost always available to give advice. As HDU beds are in short supply, seeing patients first thing in the morning greatly helps discharge decision making and theater planning.

The various postoperative complications that are commonly encountered are discussed in this chapter.

Bleeding

Superficial bleeding

Superficial venous bleeding is best controlled by digital compression and, where possible, elevation. Compression bandaging will maintain the hemostasis, but care must be taken to avoid distal constriction. Compression is difficult in the neck and groin, and where a significant hematoma is encountered, re-exploration of the wound, usually under general anesthetic, is required.

Bleeding from wound edges can be considerable. This is seen in both sutured wounds and in wounds left to granulate. If a pressure dressing only is used then there is a high chance that you will be called by the nursing staff half an hour later to tell you that the dressing that you so carefully applied is soaked with blood and has fallen off. If the bleeding site can be identified then insertion of one or two sutures under local anesthetic should be sufficient to arrest the hemorrhage.

Minor oozing after hemorrhoidectomy is common. If an artery is bleeding then the patient will produce approximately 100–200 mL of clotted blood into the bed pan every 15–20 minutes. When bleeding of this order is encountered a return visit to theater is required to under-run the bleeding vessel. If blood loss is dramatic, insert a catheter with the balloon blown-up and apply traction to it (to tamponade the blood loss) until theater.

Deep hemorrhage

The surgical resident is often asked to make a decision regarding the severity of bleeding on the basis of the volume of blood draining into abdominal drains, stoma bags and chest drains.

With deep hemorrhage the following questions should be answered:

- is the fluid pure blood?
- over what period of time has it accumulated?
- what is the total measured volume of fluid?
- what operation has been performed and has the surgeon commented about hemostasis?
- was an intraperitoneal wash-out performed?
- is there a bleeding tendency and/or is the patient anticoagulated?

If the fluid is pure blood and there has been a large total volume (greater than 500 mL in 12 hours) or rapid fluid accumulation (greater than 100 mL/hour), and concerns about hemostasis have been raised in the operation note, then there is excess bleeding and a more senior opinion is required. Look for the usual signs of hemorrhage; tachycardia and hypotension. Patients with significant hemorrhage are frequently agitated and have poor urine output. Blood should be sent for hemoglobin measurement, cross-matching and a clotting screen. Whether the patient ultimately requires re-operation or not, adequate fluid volumes (blood as soon as it is available) should be given to restore the blood pressure (BP) and an adequate urine output. Any sign of oliguria (less than 0.5 mL/kg/hour) suggests an urgent need to restore the circulating blood volume.

The patient with an epidural anesthetic can present a particularly difficult diagnostic challenge. In the early postoperative period (the first 24 hours) the patient may be impressively hypotensive and the surgical resident may be asked to determine whether or not this is due to hemorrhage. The patient with epidural-induced hypotension has a mild tachycardia, is calm rather than agitated, and has no external evidence of significant blood loss. The patient may have a reasonable or good urine output but note that if the renal perfusion pressure falls then urine production will decrease. The correct course of action is to check the hemoglobin level, give an appropriate fluid challenge of 500–1000 mL and make sure that the hypotension improves over the next 1–2 hours.

Before reducing the epidural rate, seek advice from the acute pain team (if available). If there is an excessively profound neural block with limb weakness or wider than necessary analgesia, then seek the advice of the anesthetist concerned or the on-call team.

Abscess

Superficial

Most wound infections are straightforward subcutaneous collections of pus. The presenting features of pain, swelling, erythema and tenderness are easily recognized, although tension in the wound may make detection of fluctuance difficult. The correct treatment is to open the wound sufficiently to drain the collection. For all but the largest collections, this can be done under no or local anesthetic, on the ward or in the minor operation room. A sufficient number of sutures are removed to allow easy egress of pus. This can often be done without opening up the entire wound. It is helpful to express any further pus by compression on the surrounding tissues. Packing is not of any great benefit and the patient should be encouraged to bathe the wound.

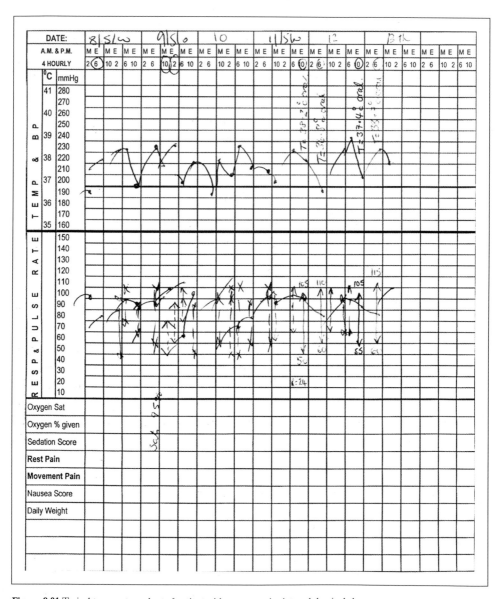

Figure 9.01 Typical temperature chart of patient with postoperative intra-abdominal abscess.

Deep abscess

An intra-abdominal abscess can occur after any laparotomy but is more likely if there was significant intraperitoneal contamination at the time of surgery. Diagnosis is more difficult than for superficial abscesses. Presentation depends on the site of collection.

Common features of an intra-abdominal abscess are:

- abdominal pain
- non-specific malaise
- anorexia
- nausea and vomiting
- failure of bowel function to return to normal with or without ileus
- a swinging pyrexia to 38°C and above, with abdominal tenderness (see Figure 9.01)
- an elevated white blood cell (WBC) count
- low or falling albumin level

In addition to the above, a subphrenic abscess is associated with a pleural effusion on the affected side. A pelvic abscess is associated with diarrhea.

Fortunately, ultrasound examination will detect the vast majority of abscesses. It is less successful in patients who have paralytic ileus, multiple drains or stomas, or when pus is confined to the pelvis. Under these circumstances, or where clinical suspicion remains high despite a normal ultrasound scan, computed tomograph (CT) scanning is the investigation of choice. WBC scanning is useful if ultrasound and CT are negative or equivocal and if clinical suspicion remains. Where technically possible, radiologists should drain deep abscesses percutaneously. It is worth remembering that if a patient has developed one intraperitoneal abscess then he or she is capable of developing another or re-accumulating pus at the same site.

Acute gastric dilatation

This rare complication can occur after any abdominal operation. The stomach becomes massively dilated and can contain over 2 L of fluid (see Figure 9.02). Complications occur because of the risk of aspiration, dehydration, deranged electrolyte levels and splinting of the diaphragm. The patient looks pale and sweaty and vomits very dark almost black watery fluid. The dilated stomach may be visible through the abdominal wall, but is sometimes masked by generalized abdominal distension. A nasogastric (NG) tube should be inserted even if the vomiting has been

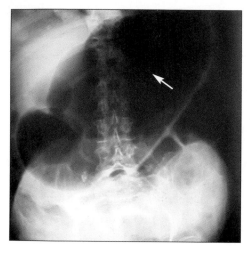

Figure 9.02 Acute gastric dilatation (arrow).

copious and you think the stomach should therefore be empty. Electrolyte levels should be checked (particularly the serum potassium and magnesium levels) and fluid and electrolyte losses should be replaced.

Postoperative arrhythmia

This is the most common postoperative complication encountered in the HDU, with atrial fibrillation being the most frequent presentation. Most junior doctors remember that the main causes of atrial fibrillation are thyrotoxicosis and ischemic heart disease.

In the postoperative patient the following causes are much more common:

- acute hypovolemia
- hypomagnesemia
- hypoxia

When faced with an acute arrhythmia:

- check the degree of hydration (pulse, BP, urine output)
- perform a full blood count (FBC)
- check urea and electrolytes (U&E)
- check calcium levels
- check magnesium levels
- check blood gases
- perform an ECG

A patient going into atrial fibrillation may well become acutely hypotensive as the atrial contribution to ventricular filling is suddenly lost. Increasing the pre-load rapidly may reverse this effect, but careful monitoring for signs of failure will be needed, preferably in a high dependency environment. Watch the fluid balance, with hourly urine output as a minimum standard.

Electrolyte abnormalities should be corrected in the first instance and this may be sufficient to correct the arrhythmia. Whether the arrhythmia is symptomatic or not, the anesthetist, resident medical officer or more senior physician should be asked for advice. This is important firstly to confirm that your interpretation of the ECG is correct and secondly because the correct medical treatment needs to address the best ways of managing the heart and not just the arrhythmia. Getting the diagnosis or treatment wrong may prove fatal.

Postoperative hypoxemia

Early postoperative hypoxemia
This is common and usually short-lived. There are many anesthetic related causes for this and the problem should be identified and a management plan formed (with the involvement of the anesthetist) prior to the patient's discharge from the recovery unit.

Late postoperative hypoxemia
Some patients remain hypoxemic or develop the problem hours or days later. It is this group that demands the close attention of the team.

How low?
Most agree that an arterial oxygen tension (pO_2) below 8 kPa (60 mmHg) constitutes postoperative hypoxemia.

Why worry?
- the risk of progression to respiratory failure
- the risk of myocardial ischemia
- it may be an early warning of sepsis and multiple organ failure
- poor gut oxygenation is prejudicial to wound and anastomotic integrity

Monitor
- pulse oximetry is commonly available, has instant read-out and is non-invasive
- low saturations (less than 94%) should lead to an arterial blood gas estimation
- always document the inspired oxygen concentration (expressed as a fraction, FiO_2) at the time of the reading or blood sampling

Some basic physiology – a reminder

Tissue oxygenation depends on blood flow and oxygen content. Flow depends on cardiac output (and local vascular resistance). Oxygen content depends on hemoglobin and oxygenation (i.e. lung function). Thus a low saturation reading from a pulse oximeter may be seen in a hypotensive, vasoconstricted patient whose respiratory component is acceptable.

Focusing on oxygenation, the cause of the problem may be:

- respiratory depression (narcotic-related?)
- reduced lung volume (reduction in functional residual capacity [FRC] is common, particularly after upper abdominal and thoracic surgery)
- chest infection
- left ventricular failure
- fluid overload

A careful clinical examination and a review of the fluid balance chart (a vital part of postoperative care) should provide the diagnosis in most cases. The simple observation of respiratory rate is most useful. While you are determining a diagnosis, give oxygen!

Oxygen therapy

!   Don't be afraid to give adequate concentrations of oxygen.

The risk of producing respiratory arrest by blocking hypoxic drive has been exaggerated in the past. As a rule of thumb, anyone who is in respiratory distress, or is hypoxemic, needs a high inspired FiO_2. However, this should be prescribed accurately in terms of concentration, flow, duration, method of administration and mode of monitoring.

Low-flow oxygen

Low-flow oxygen, given via a Hudson mask or similar, or by nasal 'spectacles', should be adequate for the mild respiratory depression associated with good narcotic-based analgesia. Patients using patient-controlled analgesia should receive low-flow oxygen for the duration of this therapy and it should be considered in any situation in which large or frequent doses of opioids are needed. (Note that failure to provide pain relief is associated with impaired lung function with shallow tidal breaths, guarding and poor compliance with physiotherapy.)

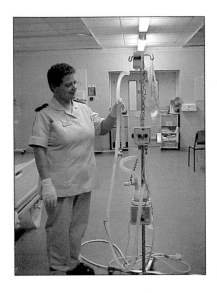

Figure 9.03 High-flow oxygen equipment.

High-flow oxygen

The apparatus used to supply high-flow oxygen comprises wide-bore tubing, an air entrainment device and a method of humidification (see Figure 9.03). Higher concentrations of oxygen are possible and the increased flow rate reduces the dilution effect of air being drawn in around the mask during peak inspiration. It is often used during the weaning process following more advanced respiratory support. Although it might suffice in some cases, it does nothing to address the underlying cause of the problem.

Continuous positive airways pressure

CPAP requires a mask that forms a seal around the face, a source of high-flow, humidified air/oxygen mix, suitable oxygen and flow failure alarms. This set-up is not available on the general wards and requires the supervision of trained HDU or ICU nurses. The essential ingredient is the raised pressure at the airway throughout both inspiration and expiration. The pressure is provided by a device of known resistance in the expiratory part of the circuit.

The effect is to increase lung volume, restoring the FRC. Closure of small airways with the attendant shunting can be reduced and collapsed airways may be re-expanded—'recruitment'. Thus, this form of therapy helps to address the cause of the problem rather than merely disguising it. A patient failing to improve or deteriorating on CPAP should be referred for possible assisted ventilation.

It is worth instituting CPAP early in the 'at-risk' group. Many of these cases can be spotted preoperatively.

The following factors increase the risk of airway closure:
- obesity
- smoking
- respiratory disease
- recumbency
- operation site (as previously noted)

Early active management in the 'at-risk' group can reduce morbidity and mortality.

Chest infection

Postoperative chest infection is very common in general surgical patients due to a combination of pre-existing respiratory disease, decreased ciliary motility following intubation and anesthesia, and reduced diaphragmatic movement secondary to postoperative pain and paralytic ileus. If general anesthetic is unavoidable in patients with co-existing respiratory disease, then respiratory complications can be reduced by good pain control, physiotherapy and oxygen therapy. Note that antibiotic prophylaxis will not prevent postoperative chest infection.

A pyrexia of around 38°C, seen in the first 24 hours after abdominal surgery, is most often due to basal atelectasis and is associated with basal crepitations. Atelectasis will usually resolve with physiotherapy and oxygen. Be obsessive about trying to obtain sputum cultures to confirm infection and guide antibiotic therapy.

Early CPAP can help 'recruit' alveoli, whereas oxygen therapy alone may 'wallpaper over the cracks'. Obese, supine smokers typically benefit. Try to encourage an upright posture, early sitting out of bed and mobilization where possible.

Antibiotic therapy is sensible for respiratory complication in the postoperative period if:
(a) atelectasis worsens or does not resolve with physiotherapy
(b) there are signs of active chest infection in patients with co-existing respiratory disease
(c) there is evidence of consolidation
(d) there is evidence of chest infection with respiratory compromise (increased respiratory rate or abnormal blood gases)
(e) sputum cultures are positive

Monitor

- respiratory rate in all patients
- blood gases in patients in categories a–d
- chest x-ray in patients in categories a and b, and in any patient who has had a thoracotomy
- continuous pulse oximetry is also useful in any patient with respiratory compromise
- consider early referral to the HDU

Respiratory failure is suspected when the respiratory rate is increasing to between 30–40/minute, when pO_2 is falling or when the carbon dioxide pressure (pCO_2) is rising. Once these criteria exist, anesthetic advice is needed and mechanical ventilation is likely to be required.

Remember that a patient is capable of talking to you even when his or her respiratory rate is 40/minute, the pO_2 is around 50 mmHg and he or she is close to respiratory arrest. Try to assess whether the patient looks tired. One of the most common scenarios is that the work of breathing becomes so great that the patient becomes exhausted. Decompensation with falling pO_2 and rising pCO_2 is then very rapid; hence the need to recognize the danger signs and intervene before decompensation occurs.

Danger signs of respiratory failure

- respiratory rate greater than 30/minute
- patient showing signs of exhaustion
- falling pO_2
- rising pCO_2

Ward management

- physiotherapy, oxygen therapy, antibiotics
- monitoring – respiratory rate, oximetry and blood gases
- HDU management – as above plus high-flow oxygen, CPAP and an arterial line
- ICU management – mechanical ventilation

Venous thrombosis and pulmonary embolus

Given that appropriate preventative measures are used with intra-operative calf compression thromboembolism deterrent stockings and subcutaneous heparin, these postoperative complications should be rare. Make sure you know what the unit policy on deep vein thrombosis (DVT) prophylaxis is, and stick to it. Clinical trials with DVT prophylaxis have shown that the main benefit is in reducing the risk of fatal postoperative pulmonary emboli.

Many small calf vein thromboses are subclinical; larger thromboses will present with calf swelling and discomfort. Any unilateral leg swelling (in a non-operated limb) should be assumed to be secondary to thrombosis unless proved otherwise. Duplex ultrasound scanning is non-invasive and accurate and should be used to confirm the diagnosis. Controversy exists about the necessity of treating calf vein thromboses. If there are no contraindications to anticoagulation, the risks from subcutaneous therapeutic low-molecular-weight heparin therapy (which does not require monitoring) and 3-month oral anticoagulation are small. All thromboses more proximal than the calf should be treated.

The classical presentation of pulmonary embolus occurs about a week postoperatively. The patient who was making a straightforward recovery from surgery develops a sudden onset of dyspnea with variable pleuritic chest pain, tachycardia and hypotension. On examination the patient is usually pale and sweaty with a raised respiratory rate. The chest examination may be otherwise normal: palpate for tenderness and auscultate for a rub (particularly at the site of pain or tenderness). Look for signs of respiratory failure and examine the abdomen to check that the patient has not developed an abdominal catastrophe.

Perform an ECG and check blood gases. The ECG is more useful for excluding a myocardial infarct than in helping to diagnose a pulmonary embolus.

In over 90% of patients with a pulmonary embolus the blood gases on air will show low pO_2.

The following questions should be answered:

(a) has the patient an acute respiratory problem?

(b) can a pulmonary embolus confidently be excluded?

(c) is there an abdominal catastrophe?

If the answer to (a) is yes, and the answers to (b) and (c) are no, then the patient should be anticoagulated. This should be initiated as soon as these questions have been answered. A ventilation perfusion scan should then be arranged. It is sensible to defer oral anticoagulation until this has been arranged but not to defer treatment with heparin.

Postoperative sepsis

In a recent article on fatal and life-threatening septic intra-abdominal complications after antireflux surgery[1] the cardinal features observed in all patients were determined.

The cardinal features of postoperative sepsis are:

• severe abdominal pain

• fever

• hypotension

• respiratory difficulties

It was noted in this article that there were often delays of several days between the beginning of alarming symptoms and intervention and that delays in treatment increased the morbidity and risk of death.

These cardinal features of life-threatening intra-abdominal sepsis are the same after gastric, hepato-biliary, pancreatic, small intestinal and colorectal surgery. The timing of these complications is most often several days after surgery when abdominal and wound pain are improving. Thus, acute deterioration and pain should alert you to the possibility of intra-abdominal complications. The development of hypotension and low urine output may simply be due to inadequate fluid input, but is worrying when combined with abdominal pain and when BP is not easily restored with fluid replacement.

In a review article on the management of septic shock, Dr JD Edwards[2] stated: "I cannot overemphasise the importance of tachypnea as a presenting clinical feature of septic shock or the value of regular assessment of respiratory rate and pattern during treatment." When assessing these patients, look at the operation note to predict the likely site of the sepsis. Determine the degree of abdominal tenderness, pulse, BP, respiratory rate and urine output.

[1]Rantanen T, Salo J, Sipponen J. Fatal and life-threatening complications in antireflux surgery: analysis of 5502 operations. Br J Surg 1999;86:1573–7.

[2]Edwards JD. Management of septic shock. BMJ 1993;306:1661–4.

Measure

- FBC
- U&E
- glucose
- ECG
- CXR
- blood gases

Management

- oxygen – monitor oxygen saturation using pulse oximetry and repeat blood gas measurements
- intravenous fluid therapy – this is guided by changes in BP, pulse, respiratory rate and urine output. The volume of fluid given is more important than whether it is crystalloid or colloid
- broad-spectrum antibiotics – remember that the patient will often already have had prophylactic and therapeutic antibiotics. The drug given should be at least as broad-spectrum as that given previously and it is usually worthwhile giving a different antibiotic. Prior to treatment take cultures including blood cultures

Response to therapy is judged by increases in BP, arterial oxygen saturation and urine output, and decreases in respiratory rate and pulse. Avoid the temptation to give vasopressor therapy (dopamine, dobutamine or adrenaline) to improve the BP. This treatment must only be carried out in the ICU with appropriate monitoring. With appropriate therapy, improvements should be seen within a few hours. If this does not occur the patient needs to be moved to the HDU or ICU and the case discussed with the senior surgical staff and the ICU staff. The HDU is not in itself a treatment so, whilst monitoring is more intensive, the patient still needs active treatment.

In a patient who is not responding to ward or HDU therapy, blood gases will typically show:

- low pH
- low arterial pO_2
- normal arterial pCO_2
- increased blood lactate concentration

With this combination, respiratory rates are usually around 30–40/minute and the patient is near to death. Transfer to the ICU is required urgently. In most patients the

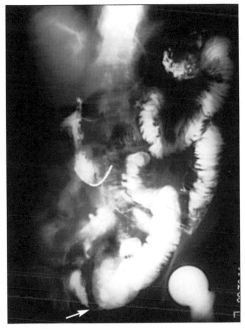

Figure 9.04 Postoperative mechanical small bowel obstruction identified by a small bowel enema (arrow).

resuscitative measures are more important than radiological tests. As long as the patient is stable and improving, ultrasound examination with drainage of collections or contrast studies to determine anastomotic integrity are possible and useful. In more seriously ill patients, this will not be possible and a senior opinion is needed to determine whether re-operation is required.

Postoperative ileus

Following intra-abdominal surgery, restoration of fluid and food intake does not usually begin until the return of peristaltic activity in the GI tract. Clinically this is assessed by a combination of reduction in the NG aspirate (when a NG tube has been inserted), improvement in abdominal distension, and the passage of flatus and stool. The return of normal GI function in most patients takes 3–4 days with a range of 1–7 days.

A postoperative ileus is diagnosed when NG aspirates remain high or the patient vomits with abdominal distension in the absence of bowel sounds and flatus. If there are no intra-abdominal complications causing the ileus, such as an abscess or electrolyte disturbances, it will resolve in 2–4 days. Thus, by 7–8 days after surgery, normal bowel function will have been restored even when the surgery has been

131

complicated by ileus. If this has not occurred by this time then mechanical rather than functional small bowel obstruction should be considered. Mechanical small bowel obstruction is more likely if the bowel has begun to work and the patient has passed flatus or stool and then stops again.

If there are clinical features of an abscess, ultrasound or CT scanning are valuable. Plain x-rays merely show distended loops of small bowel and the key question that needs to be answered is whether or not the bowel is patent. Contrast radiology is increasingly used to answer this question with either barium or gastrografin used as the contrast medium (see Figure 9.04). If there is then a complete obstruction, laparotomy is required. If contrast does pass into the colon then a further period of conservative therapy is usually appropriate. Making a decision to operate purely on clinical ground without contrast studies will result in some patients having an unnecessary laparotomy.

Abbreviations

A&E	accident and emergency
AAA	abdominal aortic aneurysm
APACHE	Acute Physiology and Chronic Health Evaluation
ASA	American Society of Anesthesiologists
BO	bowel opening
BP	blood pressure
CPAP	continuous positive airway pressure
CT	computed tomography
CVP	central venous pressure
CXR	chest x-ray
DVT	deep vein thrombosis
ECG	electrocardiogram
ERC	endoscopic retrograde cholangiography
ERCP	endoscopic retrograde cholangiopancreatography
EUA	examined under anesthesia
FBC	full blood count
FRC	functional residual capacity
GI	gastrointestinal
GMC	General Medical Council
GP	general practitioner
Hb	hemoglobin
HDU	high dependency unit
HST	higher surgical trainee
ICU	intensive care unit
ISQ	in status quo
ITU	intensive therapy unit
IU	international unit
IV	intravenous
IVU	intravenous urography
KUB	kidney, ureter and bladder (scan)
LFT	liver function test
MI	myocardial infarction
MSOF	multiple system organ failure
MSU	mid-stream urine

NG	nasogastric
pCO2	carbon dioxide pressure
pO2	oxygen tension
POSSUM	Physiological and Operative Severity Score for the enUmeration of Mortality and Morbidity
PSA	prostate specific antigen
PUJ	pelvi-ureteric junction
PR	per rectal
U&E	urea and electrolytes
USS	ultrasound scan
UTI	urinary tract infection
WBC	white blood cell

Index